Yoga: A Practical Approach

Yoga: A Practical Approach

Maeve White

STATES
ACADEMIC PRESS
www.statesacademicpress.com

Yoga: A Practical Approach
Maeve White
ISBN: 978-1-63989-574-8 (Hardback)

Published by States Academic Press,
109 South 5th Street,
Brooklyn, NY 11249, USA

Cataloging-in-Publication Data

Yoga : a practical approach / Maeve White.
p. cm.
Includes bibliographical references and index.
ISBN 978-1-63989-574-8
1. Yoga. 2. Yoga--Therapeutic use. 3. Yoga--Physiological aspects. I. White, Maeve.
RM727.Y64 Y64 2022
613.704 6--dc23

For more information regarding States Academic Press and its products, please visit the publisher's website www.statesacademicpress.com

Table of Contents

	Preface	**VII**
Chapter 1	**Yoga and its Poses**	**1**
	a. History of Yoga	1
	b. Fundamentals of Yoga Sadhna	3
	c. Health Benefits of Yoga	5
	d. Types of Yoga Poses	7
Chapter 2	**Branches of Yoga**	**36**
	a. Raja Yoga	36
	b. Hatha Yoga	40
	c. Jnana Yoga	42
	d. Karma Yoga	46
	e. Bhakti Yoga	52
	f. Tantra Yoga	58
	g. Mantra Yoga	61
Chapter 3	**Yoga Physiology and Doctrine**	**66**
	a. Yoga Physiology	66
	b. Three Bodies Doctrine	69
	c. Kosha	72
	d. Chakra	74
	e. Nadi	85
Chapter 4	**Techniques of Yoga**	**89**
	a. Anuyoga	89
	b. Mahayoga	92
	c. Sahaja Yoga	96
	d. Asana	100
	e. Mudra	105
	f. Kriyā	114
	g. Yamas	117
	h. Niyama	119
	i. Pratyahara	125
Chapter 5	**Pranayama and its Types**	**129**
	a. Bhastrika Pranayama	140
	b. Anuloma Pranayama	143
	c. Bhramari Pranayama	149
	d. Bahya Pranayama	151

Chapter 6 **Shatkarma: Yoga Cleansing Techniques** **155**
a. Neti 157
b. Dhauti 163
c. Nauli 167
d. Basti 171
e. Kapalabhati 176
f. Trataka 185

Chapter 7 **Yoga in Religion** **194**
a. Yoga and Hinduism 194
b. Yoga and Jainism 213
c. Yoga and Buddhism 224

Permissions

Index

Preface

Yoga refers to a group of mental, physical and spiritual practices which originated in ancient India. It is a spiritual science which aims to bring harmony between the mind and body. Physical activities in yoga consist of asanas which are accompanied by breathing exercises. They usually end with relaxation and meditation. Yogic exercises are broadly classified into hath yoga, raja yoga and tantric yoga. Hath yoga focuses primarily on building physical and mental strength using exercises and postures. Practices of yoga also find their roots in various religions such as Buddhism and Jainism. Regular practice of yoga improves medical conditions, lowers stress and promotes relaxation. The topics included in this book on yoga are of utmost significance and bound to provide incredible insights to readers. Some of the diverse topics covered herein, address the varied branches that fall under this category. For someone with an interest and eye for detail, this book covers the most significant topics in the field of yoga.

Given below is the chapter wise description of the book:

Chapter 1- Yoga refers to a set of mental, physical and spiritual practices which focus on controlling and stilling the mind. It comprises of various poses which have different health benefits. This chapter has been carefully written to provide a brief introduction to the varied facets of yoga such as the different types of yogic poses and the fundamentals of yoga sadhna.

Chapter 2- Some of the prominent branches of yoga are hatha yoga, raja yoga, jnana yoga, karma yoga, bhakti yoga, tantra yoga and mantra yoga. Hatha yoga is the branch of yoga which is used as a form of physical exercise. This chapter closely examines these key branches of yoga to provide an extensive understanding of the subject.

Chapter 3- The human body within the domain of yoga is considered to be composed of five koshas, or sheaths. It also comprises energy channels which can be influenced and stimulated through yoga practice. The topics elaborated in this chapter will help in gaining a better perspective about the different aspects of human body in yoga such as kosha, chakra and nadi.

Chapter 4- There are various practices and techniques which are an integral part of yoga such as anuyoga, mahayoga, sahaja yoga, asana, mudra, kriyi, yamas, niyama and pratyahara. The aim of this chapter is to explore these practices and techniques of yoga. These topics are crucial for a complete understanding of the subject.

Chapter 5- The practice within yoga which focuses on breathing is known as pranayama. It involves complete suspension of breathing. Some of the major forms of pranayama are bhastrika pranayama, anuloma pranayama, bahya pranayama and bhramari pranayama. This chapter discusses in detail these forms of pranayama.

Chapter 6- The set of practices within hatha yoga which aim at purifying the body in order to prepare a person for moksha, or liberation, is known as shatkarma. These practices include neti, dhauti, nauli, basti, kapalabhati and trataka. The topics elaborated in this chapter will help in gaining a better perspective about these purification techniques used in yoga.

Chapter 7- In addition to being a set of physical and mental practices, yoga also comprises religious practices. It is an integral aspect of various religions in the Indian subcontinent such as Hinduism, Jainism and Buddhism. This chapter closely examines the relationship of yoga with these religions as well as its depiction in popular culture in order to provide an extensive understanding of the subject.

At the end, I would like to thank all those who dedicated their time and efforts for the successful completion of this book. I also wish to convey my gratitude towards my friends and family who supported me at every step.

Maeve White

1

Yoga and its Poses

Yoga refers to a set of mental, physical and spiritual practices which focus on controlling and stilling the mind. It comprises of various poses which have different health benefits. This chapter has been carefully written to provide a brief introduction to the varied facets of yoga such as the different types of yogic poses and the fundamentals of yoga sadhna.

Yoga is essentially a spiritual discipline based on an extremely subtle science, which focuses on bringing harmony between mind and body. It is an art and scince of healthy living. The word 'Yoga' is derived from the Sanskrit root 'Yuj', meaning 'to join' or 'to yoke' or 'to unite'. As per Yogic scriptures the practice of Yoga leads to the union of individual consciousness with that of the Universal Consciousness, indicating a perfect harmony between the mind and body, Man & Nature. According to modern scientists, everything in the universe is just a manifestation of the same quantum firmament. One who experiences this oneness of existence is said to be in yoga, and is termed as a yogi, having attained to a state of freedom referred to as mukti, nirvana or moksha. Thus the aim of Yoga is Self-realization, to overcome all kinds of sufferings leading to 'the state of liberation' (Moksha) or 'freedom' (Kaivalya). Living with freedom in all walks of life, health and harmony shall be the main objectives of Yoga practice. "Yoga" also refers to an inner science comprising of a variety of methods through which human beings can realize this union and achieve mastery over their destiny. Yoga, being widely considered as an 'immortal cultural outcome' of Indus Saraswati Valley civilization – dating back to 2700 B.C., has proved itself catering to both material and spiritual upliftment of humanity. Basic humane values are the very identity of Yoga Sadhana.

History of Yoga

The science of yoga has its origin thousands of years ago, long before the first religions or belief systems were born. In the yogic lore, Shiva is seen as the first yogi or Adiyogi, and the first Guru or Adi Guru.

Several Thousand years ago, on the banks of the lake Kantisarovar in the Himalayas, Adiyogi poured his profound knowledge into the legendary Saptarishis or "seven sages". The sages carried this powerful yogic science to different parts of the world, including Asia, the Middle East, Northern Africa and South America. Interestingly, modern scholars have noted and marvelled at the close parallels found between ancient cultures across the globe. However, it was in India that the yogic system found its fullest expression. Agastya, the Saptarishi who travelled across the Indian subcontinent, crafted this culture around a core yogic way of life.

A number of seals and fossil remains of Indus Saraswati valley civilization with Yotic motives and figures performing yoga indicate the presence of Yoga in India. The Number of seals and fossil remains of Indus Saraswati valley civilization with Yogic motives and figures performing Yoga Sadhana suggest the presence of Yoga in ancient India. The phallic symbols, seals of idols of mother Goddess are suggestive of Tantra Yoga. Presence of Yoga is available in folk traditions, Indus valley civilization, Vedic and Upanishadic heritage, Buddhist and Jain traditions, Darshanas, epics of Mahabharat and Ramayana, theistic traditions of Shaivas, Vaishnavas, and Tantric traditions. In addition, there was a primordial or pure Yoga which has been manifested in mystical traditions of South Asia. This was the time when Yoga was being practised under the direct guidance of Guru and its spritual value was given special importance. It was a part of Upasana and yoga sadhana was inbuilt in their rituals. Sun was given highest importance during the vedic period. The practice of 'Surya namaskara' may have been invented later due to this influence. Pranayama was a part of daily ritual and to offer the oblation. Though Yoga was being practiced in the pre-Vedic period, the great Sage Maharshi Patanjali systematized and codified the then existing practices of Yoga, its meaning and its related knowledge through his Yoga Sutras. After Patanjali, many Sages and Yoga Masters contributed greatly for the preservation and development of the field through their well documented practices and literature.

Historical evidences of the existence of Yoga were seen in the pre-vedic period (2700 B.C.), and thereafter till Patanjali's period. The main sources, from which we get the information about Yoga practices and the related literature during this period, are available in Vedas (4), Upanishads(108), Smritis, teachings of Buddhism, Jainism, Panini, Epics (2), Puranas (18) etc.

Tentatively, the period between 500 BC - 800 A.D. is considered as the Classical period which is also considered as the most fertile and prominent period in the history and development of Yoga. During this period, commentaries of Vyasa on Yoga Sutras and Bhagawadgita etc. came into existence. This period can be mainly dedicated to two great religious teachers of India –Mahavir and Buddha. The concept of Five great vows – Pancha mahavrata- by Mahavir and Ashta Magga or eightfold path by Buddha - can be well considered as early nature of Yoga sadhana. We find its more explicit explanation in Bhagawadgita which has elaborately presented the concept of Gyan yoga, Bhakti yoga and Karma Yoga. These three types of yoga are still the highest example of human wisdom and and even today people find peace by following the methods as shown in Gita. Patanjali's yoga sutra besides containing various aspects of yoga, is mainly identified with eight fold path of Yoga. The very important commentary on Yoga sutra by Vyasa was also written. During this very period the aspect of mind was given importance and it was clearly brought out through Yoga sadhana, Mind and body both can be brought under control to experience equanimity. The period between 800 A.D. - 1700 A.D. has been recognized as the Post Classical period wherein the teachings of great Acharyatrayas-Adi Shankracharya, Ramanujacharya, Madhavacharya-were prominent during this period. The teachings of Suradasa, Tulasidasa, Purandardasa, Mirabai were the great contributors during this period. The Natha Yogis of Hathayoga Tradition like Matsyendaranatha, Gorkshanatha, Cauranginatha, Swatmaram Suri, Gheranda, Shrinivasa Bhatt are some of the great personalities who popularized the Hatha Yoga practices during this period.

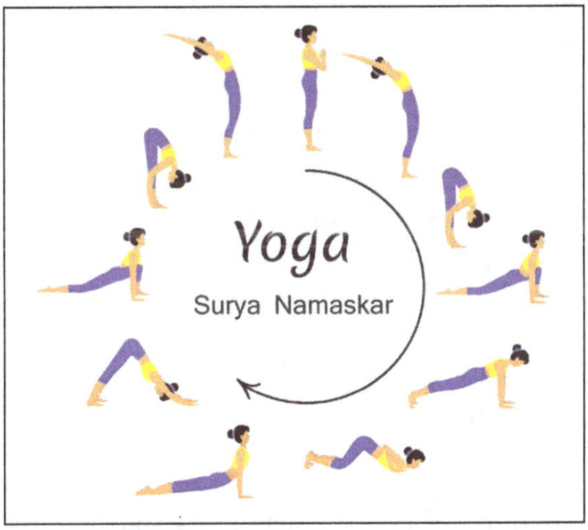

The period between 1700 - 1900 A.D. is considered as Modern period in which the great Yogacharyas- Ramana Maharshi, Ramakrishna Paramhansa, Paramhansa Yogananda, Vivekananda etc. have contributed for the development of Raja Yoga. This was the period when Vedanta, Bhakti yoga, Nathayoga or Hatha-yoga flourished. The Shadanga-yoga of Gorakshashatakam, Chaturanga-yoga of Hathayogapradipika, Saptanga-yoga of Gheranda Samhita, were the main tenents of Hatha-yoga.

Now in the contemporary times, everybody has conviction about yoga practices towards the preservation, maintenance and promotion of health. Yoga has spread all over the world by the teachings of great personalities like Swami Shivananda, Shri T.Krishnamacharya, Swami Kuvalayananda, Shri Yogendara, Swami Rama, Sri Aurobindo, Maharshi Mahesh Yogi, Acharya Rajanish, Pattabhijois, BKS. Iyengar, Swami Satyananda Sarasvati and the like.

Fundamentals of Yoga Sadhna

Systems of Yoga

Yoga works on the level of one's body, mind, emotion and energy. This has given rise to four broad classifications of Yoga: karma yoga, where we utilize the body; bhakti yoga, where we utilize the emotions; gyana yoga, where we utilize the mind and intelect; and kriya yoga, where we utilize the energy.

Each system of Yoga we practice would fall within the gamut of one or more of these categories. Every individual is a unique combination of these four factors. "All the ancient commentaries on Yoga have stressed that it is essential to work under the direction of a Guru." The reason being that only a Guru can mix the appropriate combination of the four fundamental paths, as is necessary for each seeker.

Yoga Education

Traditionally, Yoga Education was imparted by knowledgeable, experienced, and wise persons in the families (comparable with the education imparted in convents in the west) and then by the Seers (Rishis/Munis/Acharyas) in Ashramas (compared with monastries). Yoga Education, on the other hand, aims at taking care of the individual, the 'Being'. It is presumed that a good, balanced, integrated, truthful, clean, transparent person will be more useful to oneself, family, society, nation, nature and humanity at large. Yoga education is 'Being oriented'. Details of working with 'being oriented' aspect have been outlined in various living traditions and texts and the method contributing to this important field is known as 'Yoga'.

Present days, Yoga Education is being imparted by many eminent Yoga Institutions, Yoga Colleges, Yoga Universites, Yoga Departments in the Universities, Naturopathy colleges and Private trusts & societies. Many Yoga Clinics, Yoga Therapy and Training Centers, Preventive Health Care Units of Yoga, Yoga Research Centers etc. have been established in Hospitals, Dispensories, Medical Institiutions and Therapetical setups.

Chakras

The word "chakra" literally means spinning wheel. Yoga maintains that chakras are center points of energy, thoughts, feelings, and the physical body. According to yogic teachers, chakras determine the way people experience reality through emotional reactions, desires or aversions, levels of confidence or fear, and even physical symptoms and effects. When energy becomes blocked in a chakra, it is said to trigger physical, mental, or emotional imbalances that manifest in symptoms, such as anxiety, lethargy, or poor digestion.

Asanas are the many physical positions in Hatha yoga. People who practice yoga use asanas to free energy and stimulate an imbalanced chakra. There are seven major chakras, each with their own focus:

- Sahasrara: The "thousand-petaled" or "crown" chakra represents the state of pure consciousness. This chakra is located at the crown of the head, and the color white or violet represents it. Sahasrara involves matters of inner wisdom and physical death.

- Ajna: The "command" or "third-eye chakra" is a meeting point between two important energetic streams in the body. Ajna corresponds to the colors violet, indigo, or deep blue, though traditional yoga practitioners describe it as white. The ajna chakra relates to the pituitary gland, which drives growth and development.
- Vishuddha: The color red or blue represents the "especially pure" or "throat" chakra. Practitioners consider this chakra to be the home of speech, hearing, and metabolism.
- Anahata: The "unstruck" or "heart" chakra relates to the colors green and pink. Key issues involving anahata include complex emotions, compassion, tenderness, unconditional love, equilibrium, rejection, and wellbeing.
- Manipura: Yellow represents the "jewel city" or "navel" chakra. Practitioners connect this chakra with the digestive system, as well as personal power, fear, anxiety, developing opinions, and tendencies towards an introverted personality.
- Svadhishthana: Practitioners claim that the "one's own base" or "pelvic" chakra is the home of the reproductive organs, the genitourinary system, and the adrenal gland.
- Muladhara: The "root support" or "root chakra" is at the base of the spine in the coccygeal region. It is said to contain our natural urges relating to food, sleep, sex, and survival, as well as the source of avoidance and fear.

Health Benefits of Yoga

General Benefits

The benefits of various yoga techniques have been professed to improve body flexibility, performance, stress reduction, attainment of inner peace, and self-realization. The system has been advocated as a complementary treatment to aid healing of several ailments such as coronary heart disease, depression, anxiety disorders, asthma, and extensive rehabilitation for disorders including musculoskeletal problems and traumatic brain injury. The system has also been suggested as behavioral therapy for smoking cessation and substance abuse (including alcohol abuse).

- Physical:
    - Improved body flexibility and balance.

    - Improved cardiovascular endurance (stronger heart).
    - Improved digestion.
    - Improved abdominal strength.
    - Enhanced overall muscular strength.
    - Relaxation of muscular strains.
    - Weight control.
    - Increased energy levels.
    - Enhanced immune system.
- Mental:
    - Relief of stress resulting from the control of emotions.
    - Prevention and relief from stress-related disorders.
    - Intellectual enhancement, leading to improved decision-making skills.
- Spiritual:
    - Life with meaning, purpose, and direction.
    - Inner peace and tranquility.
    - Contentment.

A word of caution about the incorrect practice of yoga is necessary at this point.

Benefits of Yoga for Special Children

- Yoga helps coordinate the activities of mind, body and emotions.
- Reduces distracted state of mind thereby building up focus and concentration.
- Improves activities of day today living to the degree which could never otherwise be achieved.
- Improves one's ability and helps one to rely on their own selves making them independent.
- Helps develop social relationships, and reduces frequency of violent emotional upsets.
- Reduces the negative traits and tendency to cause injuries to self and others.

- Develops a positive outlook improving self-confidence, self-sufficiency and sociability.
- Improves interpersonal relationships.
- Improves their loco motor skills and psycho-motor coordination.
- Reduces obesity.
- Controls drooling.
- Helps in disappearance of facial tics.
- enhanced eye-hand coordination.
- improved attention span.
- Reduces hyperactivity.
- Improves appetite and sleep.
- Improves overall health.
- Increases immunity.
- Reduces aggression.
- Reduces dependency of drugs.
- Increases the efficiency of the nervous system and thus helps in their rehabilitation.

Types of Yoga Poses

Standing Poses

A firm foundation is key to the integrity of any structure. Whether it is a building or a body, the part that contacts the earth must be strong and viable. Standing poses make us aware of our connection with the earth and teach us to be relaxed and balanced on our feet. We can then realign our foundation from the ankles, through the knees, to the pelvis and tailbone, thereby connecting the core of the body to the earth. By creating awareness of alignment, standing poses also cultivate kinesthetic intelligence—an organic understanding of how the body works and moves. This prevents us from exceeding our capacity and thereby injuring our joints. Because standing poses require us to actively engage our awareness of how we use our muscles, joints, and breath, they build both mental and physical stamina as well as discipline. And, as with all the postures, standing poses improve circulation, breathing, and energy; as the body opens, energy flows more freely, and all the body's systems work more fluidly.

Triangle (*Utthita Trikonasana*)

The pose rotates the pelvis over the thighbones, loosening the hip joints and releasing the hamstrings and adductor muscles. Rather than pulling your pelvis backward, make sure that your sacrum moves into your body, toward your abdomen. Keeping the back leg straight and grounded, lengthen from the tailbone to the crown of the head while reaching the arms wide and turning your navel gently toward your top hand.

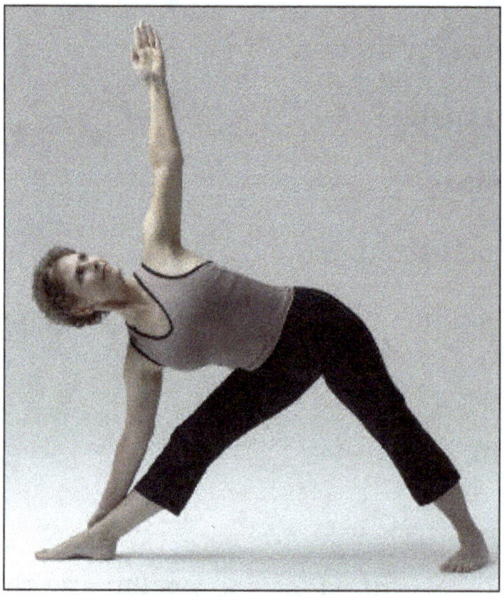

Side Angle (*Utthita Parshvakonasana*)

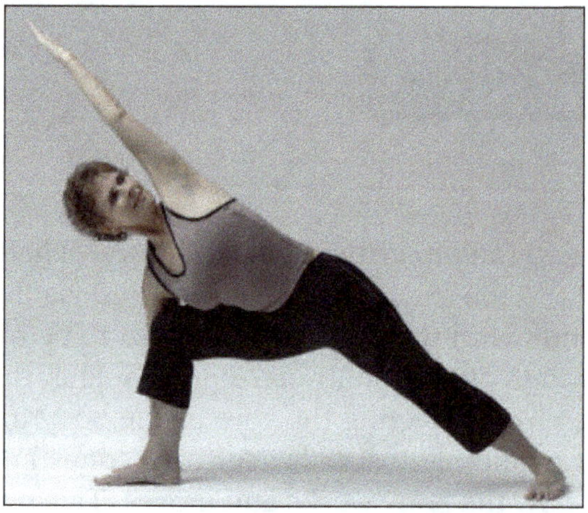

This posture is one of the most strengthening for the legs, and it helps bring balance and stability to the knee and ankle joints. The deep groin opening here feels better when the hip joints are already warm from triangle pose. The back leg is strong and weighted, the spine centered. Make sure the front knee tracks directly over the heel and ankle.

Basic Standing Forward Bend (*Uttanasana*)

After the upright standing poses, the hip joints and hamstrings are ready for a deeper forward bend, and the body is ready for a more restful pose. Bringing the head below the heart relaxes the brain and nervous system. Uttanasana can teach "right effort" as you learn to balance between effort and surrender—ideally the legs stay strong and energized while the spine and arms relax fully.

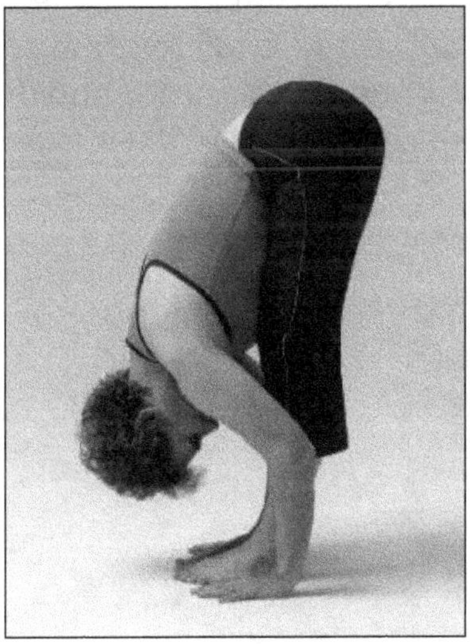

Tree Pose (*Vrikshasana*)

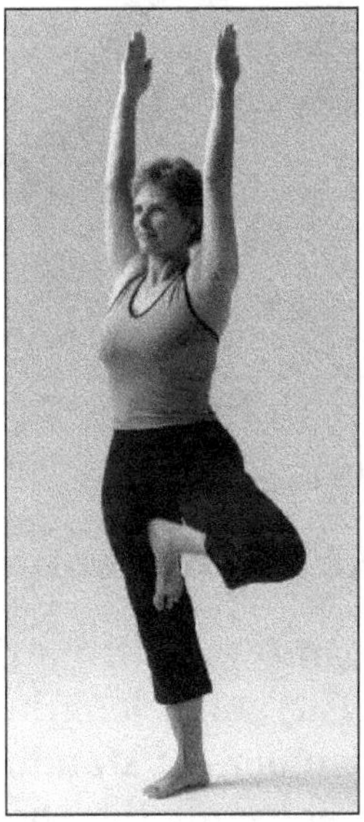

In this basic balance posture, the standing leg needs to ground strongly while the torso becomes light and the spine long. Learn to relax your shoulders as you raise your arms overhead, reaching from the back of the rib cage rather than lifting the tops of the shoulders. Keep your face and sense organs soft, and balance from your inner core as you lift gently from the floor of your pelvis.

Warrior 1 (*Virabhadrasana* 1)

Here the back leg rotates internally and the psoas muscles are lengthened as the torso turns toward the front leg, giving more spinal extension and front-body opening. Turn your back foot approximately 60 degrees toward the front foot to protect the back knee. It is important to keep the front knee aligned with the heel and ankle. The shoulders and face stay relaxed as the arms reach overhead, and the spine reaches up and out of the pelvis and grounded legs. Rotating the arms externally (so that the palms keep turning toward each other) will help keep space in the shoulders and upper back.

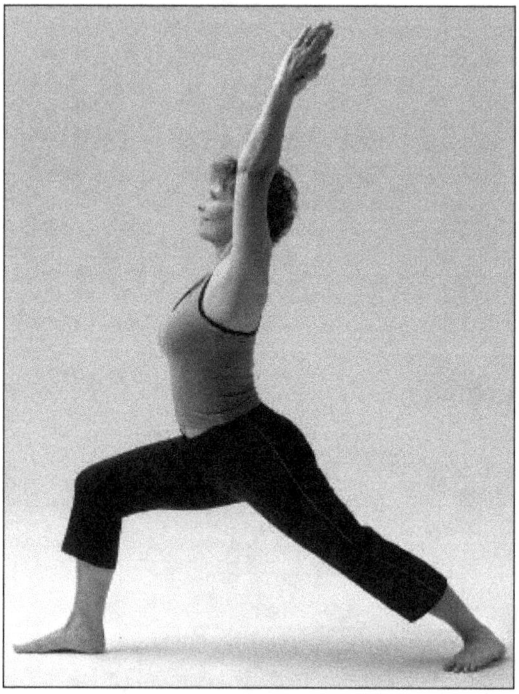

Counterposes and Cooldowns

Downward Dog (*Adho Mukha Svanasana*)

The hamstrings are already long and warm from the standing poses, so it will feel easier to ground the legs here. The spine lengthens from the crown of the head toward the tailbone. Bring the elements of standing poses into your dog pose, externally rotating the arms, gently engaging the abdominals, and energizing the legs and feet.

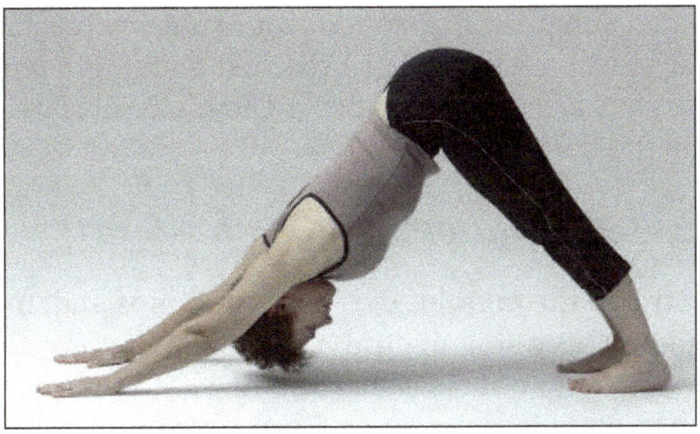

Child's Pose (*Balasana*)

This soothes the spine and the nervous system and relaxes the brain. Bring your feet toward each other, and open your knees a bit wider than your hips as you drop the pelvis down and back. Relax, letting the pelvis sink down toward the legs and the forehead rest on the floor. (If your hips are tight, fold a blanket over the calves and behind the knees, and rest the forehead on a block or on your folded arms instead of the floor.)

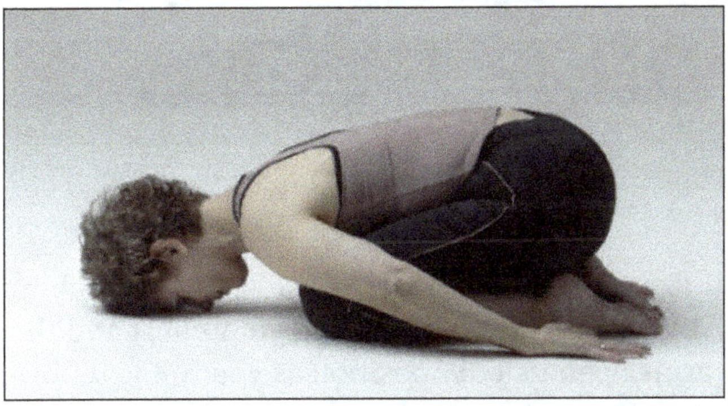

Comfortable Cross-Legged Seated Forward Bend (*Adho Mukha Sukhasana*)

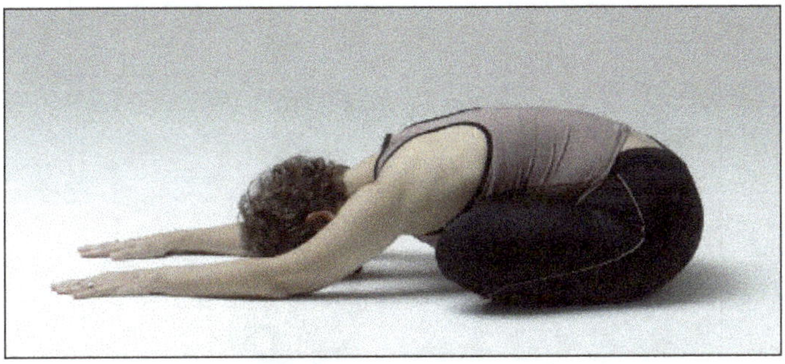

This simple forward bend is a nice counterpose for the spine; it also releases the outer hip rotators after they have worked hard to support the legs in standing poses. Keeping your sit bones grounded, lengthen the front of your spine by reaching your arms as far out in front of you as you can. Once you've reached maximum length, let your whole torso relax, including your arms and your neck. The hips will release more easily if the forehead is resting on the floor (or a block).

Reclining Leg Stretch (*Supta Padangusthasana*)

The reclining poses stretch the muscles of the legs and hips and, most important, they bring the sacroiliac joints back to a neutral, stable position. For the best results, give equal energy and awareness to both legs, lengthening both the one on the floor and the one that is stretching upward into the strap. Keep your head and shoulders relaxed as they rest on the floor.

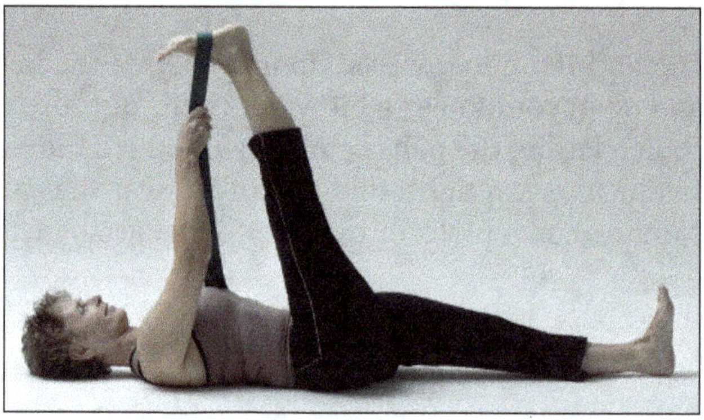

Reclining Twist

This simple version is a delicious release for the spine and the muscles of the back. Lying on your back, bring both knees up toward your chest and then drop them to the right, keeping your arms open in a "T" position as you roll your lower body gently onto your right side. Keep gently reaching back to the left with your left arm to open the belly and torso, but let gravity do most of the work here, as you feel the legs and the left arm releasing away from each other. Repeat on the other side.

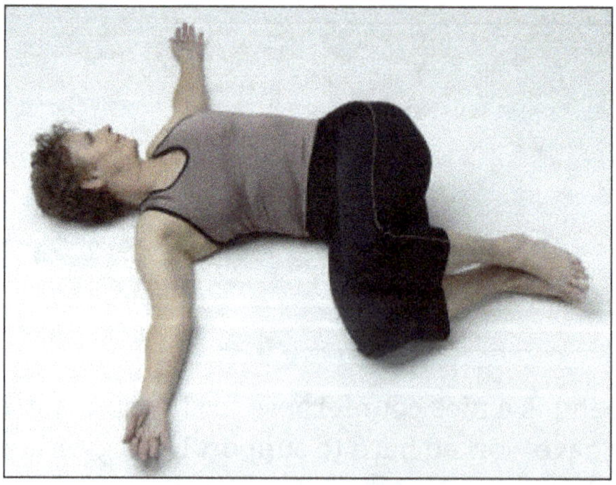

Relaxation and Integration (*Shavasana*—Five Minutes Minimum)

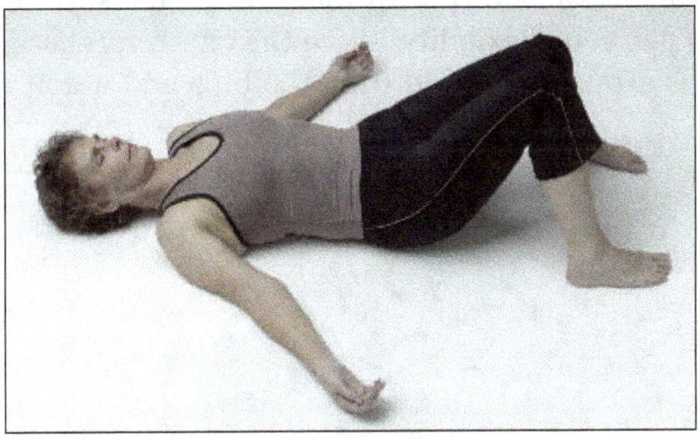

Shavasana is a key part of any practice session and should always be included. If your lower back is uncomfortable, keep your knees bent and feet flat on the floor, minimizing effort by allowing the knees to rest against one another. Another option is to place a bolster or a folded blanket under your knees.

Sitting Poses

There are sitting yoga asanas suitable for the practitioners of every level, especially the beginners or the ones who face problems doing the standing range of yoga poses. Seated yoga postures give the yoga performers the time and space to build upon their balance and flexibility. A great mind-body energizer– the sitting yoga postures work greatly on building stamina, toning the abdominal organs, massaging the internal tracts, and relieving backaches.

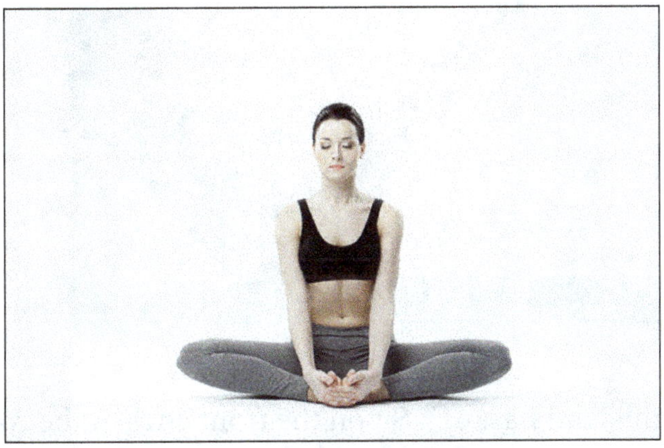

1. Bound Angle Pose (Baddha Konasana): Start this pose in a seated position on a yoga mat with legs straight in front of you. Bend the knees, pull heels close to the pelvis and drop the knees wide open to the sides with soles of the feet together. Grasp the thumbs of the feet with your fingers. Maintain the erect position throughout the pose and look in front.

2. Forward Fold (Paschimottanasana): Sit on the floor, legs unbent, and hands on the ground. Inhale and hoist the hands upward. Exhale and fold forward in one swing moving the body as one unit. Reach down with your arms and rest the hands on the ground or touch the toes as per your flexibility. Place the chest, forehead, and nose over the thighs. Keep the back straight and fold from the hips and not at the waist. Hold this pose for 60 seconds.

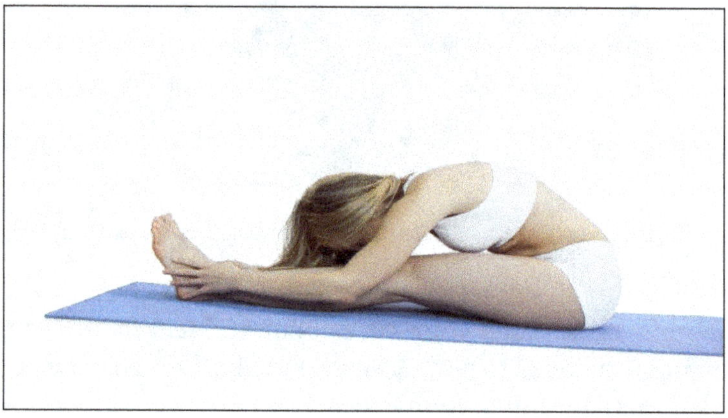

3. Boat Pose (Navasana): Begin in a staff pose (Dandasana). Take a bend at the knees and set the feet firmly on the ground. Gently lift the feet off the floor, hug the thighs into the abdomen, and lengthen the tailbone. Slowly stretch the legs out and make the shins parallel to the floor. Raise the toes slightly above the eye level. Extend the arms alongside the floor.

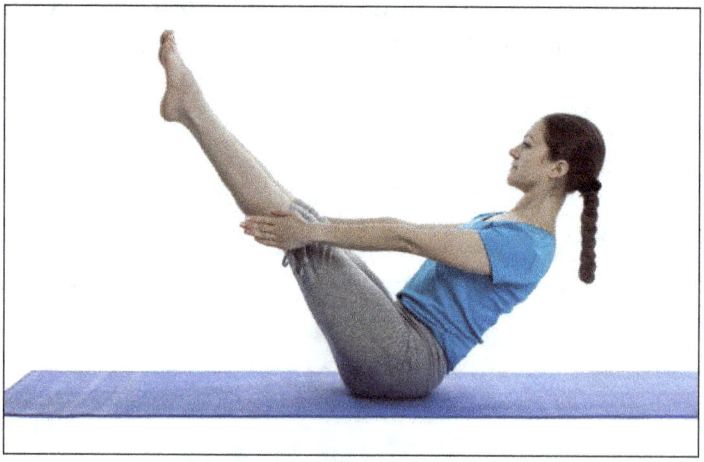

4. Fire-Log Pose (Agnistambhasana): Sit on the front edge of the yoga mat, knees folded, and feet on the mat. Roll the shoulder blades into the back and keep the head in a neutral position. Cross your legs with the right foot under the left leg to the outside of the left hip and vice-versa. Ensure the soles are perpendicular to the floor. Spread the toes and bend forward at the groins. Lay the hands on the ground in front of the shins. Repeat the same with the other leg on the top.

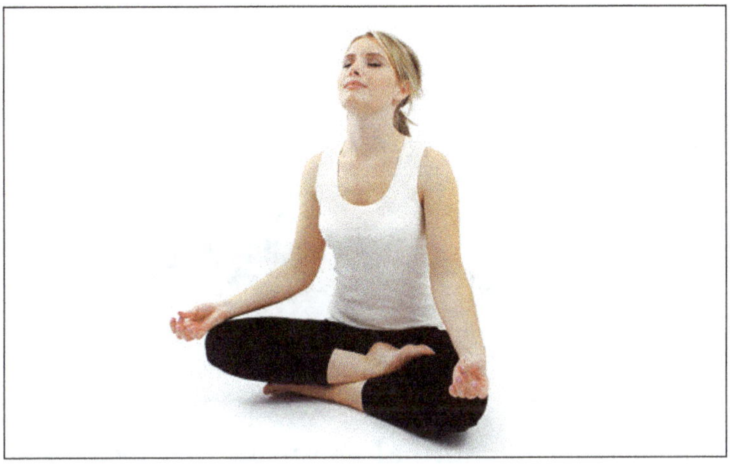

5. Head-to-Knee Forward Fold (Janu-Sirsasana): Begin this posture in a seated pose with the spine and legs straight. Breathe in and fold the right leg at the knee. Place the foot sole against the inner left thigh and heel towards the perineum. Locate the left hand beside the left hip on the floor. Extend the right hand to take the inner left foot. Now grab the outside of the foot with the left hand. Lower down and touch the thighs with your stomach and head.

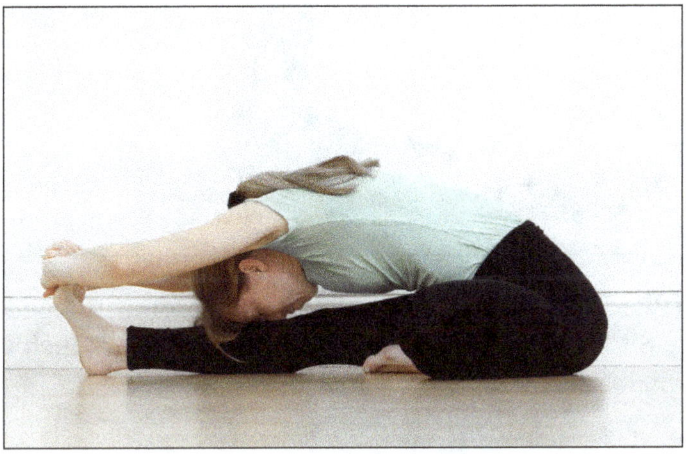

6. Hero Pose (Virasana): Come on your hands and toes with the thighs perpendicular to the ground and the inner knees touching each other. Widen the feet a little more than your hips. Turn the toes towards each other and keep the top of the feet flat on the floor. Sit back halfway with the torso leaning in the front direction moderately. Now, sit down between the feet. Hands will lay in lap or thighs, palms either up or down.

7. Easy Pose (Sukhasana): Come into a seated position with hips on the floor. Criss-Cross the legs at the shins. Place the hands on the knees in Gyan Mudra. Lengthen the body from the crown of the head to the pelvis. Draw the shoulders back and lift the chest. Relax the face and breathe.

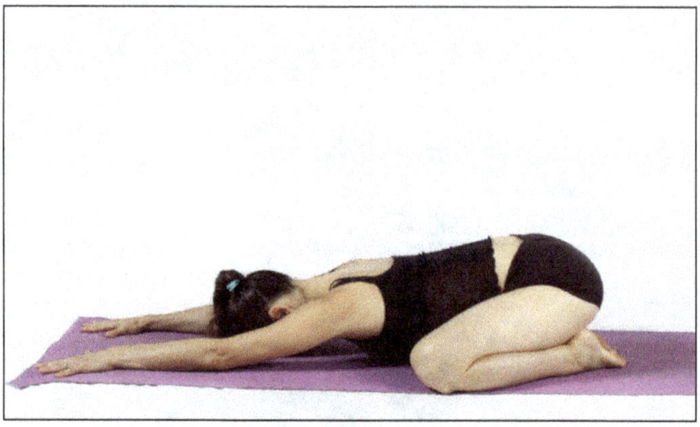

8. Staff Pose (Dandasana): Sit tall with the legs extended and together. Rotate the thighs inward and press them firmly against the floor. Keep the torso at right-angle to the floor and flex the ankles. Rest the hands beside the hips.

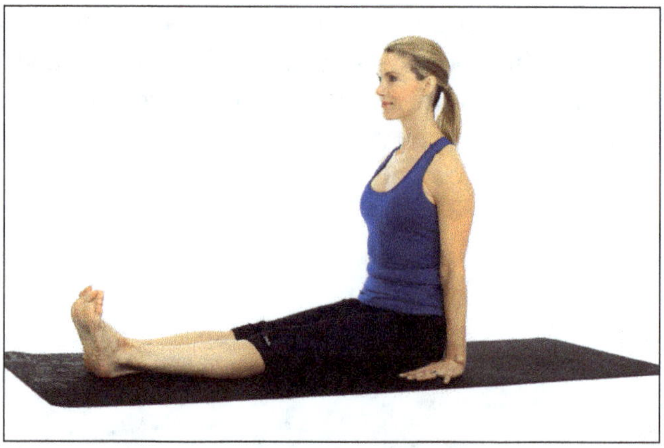

9. Gracious Pose (Bhadrasana): Start in a tabletop position with knees hip-width apart and toes touching. Sit back on the heels. Spread the knees as much as possible. Draw the shoulders down, hands on knees and chest lifted in front.

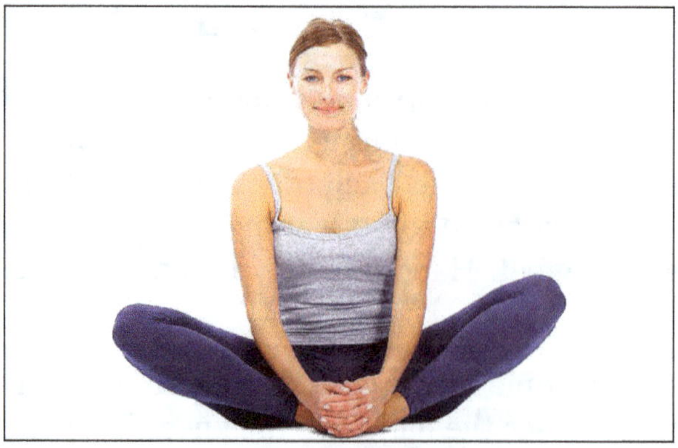

10. Lion Pose (Simhasana): Begin in a seated stance with hips resting on the heels and

palms on the knees. Exhale, bring the hands on the floor, arch the spine, and look up at the ceiling. Elongate the spine in the pose.

Kneeling Poses

When kneeling, the body's weight is on the knees, shins, and tops of the feet. Kneeling brings the center of gravity closer to the ground than standing, but farther from the ground than sitting. Kneeling, which includes both kneel-sitting and kneel-standing, is an important transitional place for babies learning to move from sitting to standing.

This position is associated with lowering oneself in the sense of meekness or worship. This probably evolved from the fact that when kneeling, a person is more vulnerable than when standing, especially if their head is bowed. Even the proud, upright stance of kings and pharaohs is tempered by their depiction in this humble position when they are at worship. Kneeling is also a posture of relaxed alertness that is associated with strength and readiness, as seen in vajrasana and virasana. In martial arts, kneeling is used as a preparatory position that is easier to stand from more quickly than sitting cross-legged, and in the practice of aikido they even train to do throws from kneeling.

In asana, kneeling poses are often used to help mobilize the hip joints. When the mobility of the feet and lower legs is removed from the base of support, attention can be focused on the actions in the hip joints, pelvic halves, and pelvic floor.

Kneeling also provides a stable and symmetrical base from which the center of gravity can be raised up so the spine can fully extend, most beautifully expressed in poses such as ustrasana and eka pada rajakapotasana.

Vajrasana

- *Thunderbolt Posture.*
- vahj-RAHS-anna.
- *vajra* = thunderbolt, diamond.

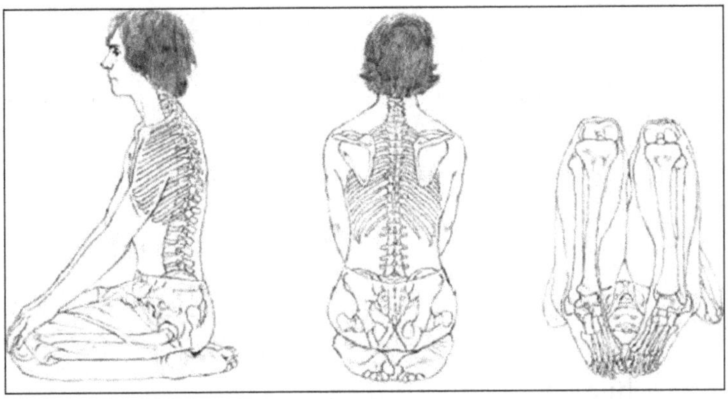

Virasana

- *Hero's Posture*
- veer-AHS-anna
- *vira* = man, hero, chief

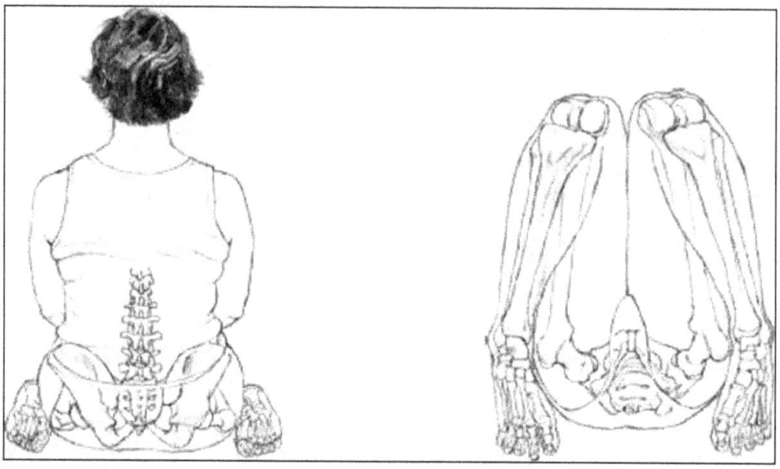

Common skeletal joint actions (for two previous poses)	
Spine	Lower limbs
Neutral or axial extension	Hip flexion, internal rotation, and abduction; knee flexion: ankle planter flexion

As in sitting poses such as sukhasana, siddhasana, and padmasana, the goal is steadiness and ease, or sthira and sukha, the fundamental qualities of all asanas as described by Patañjali in the *Yoga Sutras*. Virasasana and vajrasana are excellent poses for supporting the spine and skull in a way that allows the senses to turn inward for pranayama and meditation (like the sitting poses beginning on.

For some people, these kneeling positions are easier than sitting cross-legged because the hip joints do not need to externally rotate or adduct as they do in siddhasana or sukhasana. Kneeling poses are also more symmetrical because both legs can do the same action and neither leg is crossed in front of the other. This crossing of the legs creates an asymmetrical action in the pelvis and hips that can have long-term effects.

Balasana

- *Child's Pose.*
- bah-LAHS-anna.
- *bala* = young, childish, not fully grown or developed.

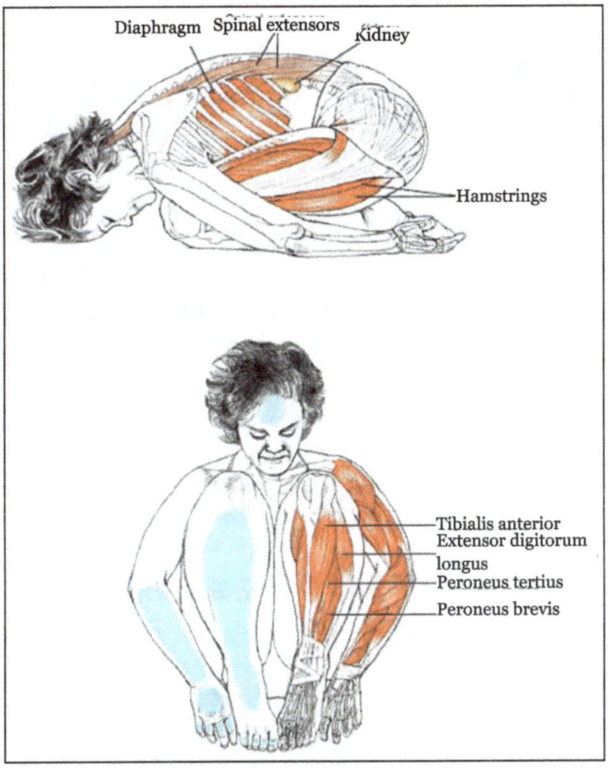

Symmetrical kneeling forward-bending pose.

Skeleton Joint Actions	
Spine	Lower limbs
Flexion	SI joint nutation, hip flexion and adduction, knee flexion, ankle planter flexion

Gravity draws the yielding body deeper into this position. One goal of this pose is to bring the sitting bones to the heels and the forehead to the floor. To do so, many muscles have to lengthen: the extensors of the spine, gluteus maximus, piriformis and other rotators, hamstrings, gluteus medius and minimus (because of hip adduction), tibialis anterior, peroneus tertius, extensor digitorum longus and brevis, and extensor hallucis longus and brevis in the feet.

Variations include widening the knees (hip abduction), which can create more neutral extension in the spine and make room for the belly; extending the arms overhead; clasping the heels with the hands; crossing the arms under the forehead; and turning the head to one side.

Sometimes there is congestion in the fronts of the hip joints. It can be caused by using the hip flexors to pull the body down toward the thighs, rather than allowing gravity to create that action. The use of props can assist in this release.

If the extensors of the toes are tight or if there is a lack of mobility in the bones of the feet, restriction can also be felt in the tops of the feet. In addition, weakness in the intrinsic muscles of the feet often results in cramping in this and similar positions.

Breathing

With the hips fully flexed and adducted and the front of the torso resting on the anterior surfaces of the thighs, the movement of the breath in the abdomen and anterior rib cage is greatly restricted. This necessitates more movement in the back of the waist and rib cage. That is why if tightness exists in those places, this pose can feel suffocating.

Supta Virasana

- *Reclining Hero Pose.*
- soup-tah veer-AHS-anna.
- *supta* = reclining, lain down to sleep; *vira* = a brave or eminent man, hero, chief.

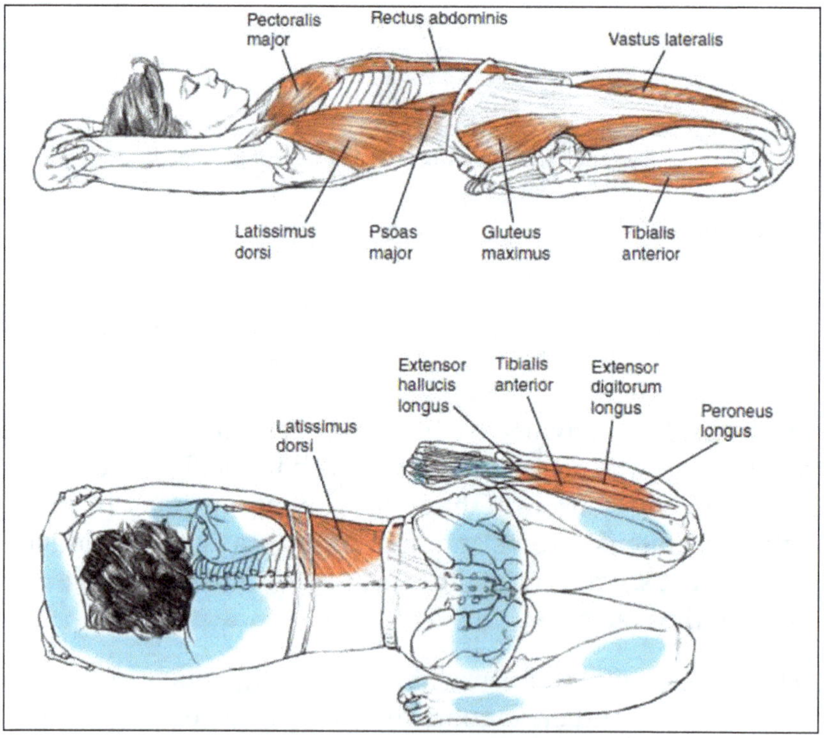

Symmetrical kneeling backward-bending pose.

Skeletal joint actions	
Spine	Lower limbs
Axial extension	SI joint counternutationi hip extension, internal rotation, and adduction: knee flexion and medial rotation: ankle planter flexion

Muscular joint actions	
Spine	
Concentric contraction	Passively lengthening
To prevent ovemobiiization of lumbar spine: Psoas minor, abdominal muscles	Psoas major
Lower limbs	
Concentric contraction	Passively lengthening
To keep knees together:	
Gracilis, adductor magnus	Psoas major, rectus femoris, vastii, sartorius, tibi- alis anterior, extensor digitorum longus, extensor hallucis longus

Many variations exist for the arm position in this pose—at the sides, reaching overhead, and propped up on the elbows. If the latissimus dorsi are short, reaching the arms overhead can cause hyperextension of the spine because of the attachment of the latissimus dorsi in the lower back.

Because hip extension in internal rotation is generally more challenging than in external rotation, supta virasana reveals how open the "groins" truly are. This pose often begins as spinal extension, especially if there is tightness in the hip flexors, because the internal rotation of the legs is bound into place by the weight of the body.

If the hip extensors are tight and the pose is forced, the force can be transmitted either into the lower back or into the knees. The pose should instead be supported in a way that allows for maximum hip extension; getting down to the floor is less important. Because the knees are at risk, keeping the feet active and avoiding supination is important for maintaining integrity in the knee joints. This can be an excellent pose for sciatic and low-back pain if done with attention to the internal rotation and extension in the hips. If poorly executed, the pose can exacerbate low-back pain.

Breathing

The tautness in the psoas major and abdominal wall creates both posterior and anterior pressure in the abdominal cavity. This effect is magnified when activating the abdominal muscles to flatten the lumbar curve. The resulting breathing patterns would favor movements above and below the abdominal pressure.

Emphasizing thoracic breath movements at the base of the rib cage helps to mobilize the upper spine and shoulder girdle. Focusing on pelvic floor movements assists in releasing tension in the hips, groins, and gluteal region.

Ustrasana

- *Camel Pose.*

- oosh-TRAHS-anna.
- *ustra* = camel.

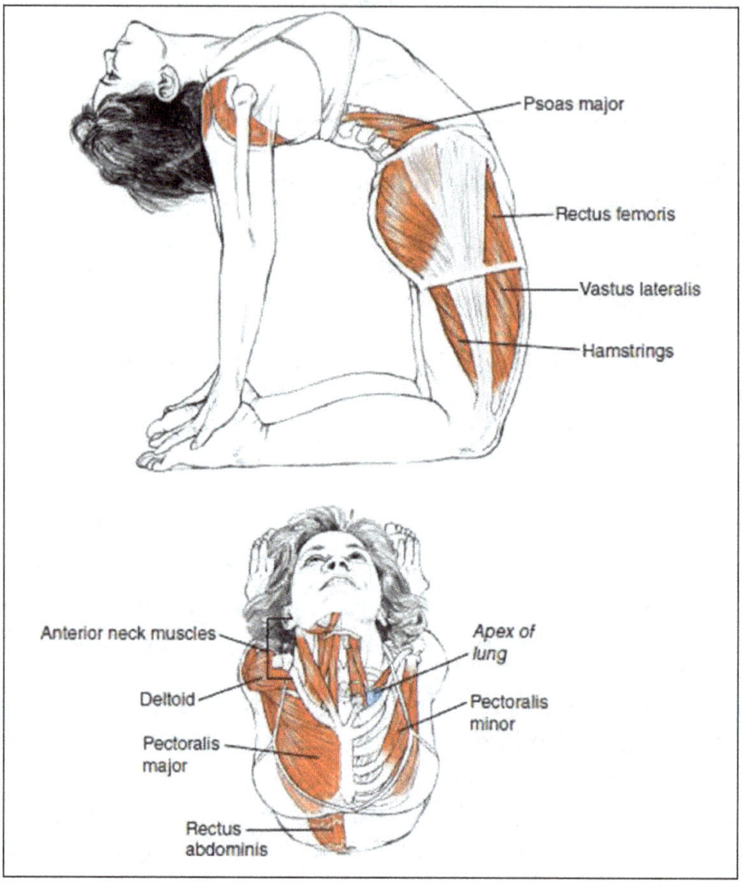

Symmetrical kneeling backward-bending pose.

Skeletal joint actions		
Spine	Upper limbs	Lower limbs
Extension	Scapular adduction and down word rotation, shoulder extension and adduction, elbow extension	SI joint counternutation, hip extension, and adduction: knee flexion and ankle planter flexion
Muscular joint action		
Spine		
Concentric contraction	Eccentric contraction	Passively lengthening
To extend spine (though most of action of extension is caused by gravity): Spinal extensors	To prevent overmobilization of Lumber spine: Psoas miner, abdominal muscles To resist hyperextension in cervical spine as head extend: Anterior neck muscles	Psoas major

Upper limbs		
Concentric contraction		Passively lengthening
To adduct, elevate. and downwardly rotate scapula: Rhomboids, levator scapulae To stabilize shoulder joint and prevent protection of head of humerus' Rotate cuff	To extend and adduct shoulder Joint: Triceps brachii (long head), teres major, posterior deltoid To extend elbow: Triceps brachii	Pectoralis major and minor, biceps brachii, Coracobrachialis
Lower limbs		
Concentric contraction	Eccentric contraction	
To extend, adduct and internally rotate hip: Hamstring, adducts Magnus, gluteus Maximus	To resist hip extortion and knee flexion: Rectus femoris To resist knee flexion: Articularis genu, vasti	

Gravity is pulling the torso into the back bend, which is checked by the arm action and the eccentric action of the spinal flexors. In the cervical spine, the anterior neck muscles are eccentrically active, but the sternocleidomastoid should not be active to avoid the base of the skull being pulled into the atlas and axis. Internal rotation of the legs will help stabilize the SI joint by encouraging the front of this joint to align.

It can be very challenging to find a healthy extension of the spine at the base of the neck or the top of the thoracic spine. It helps to focus on releasing the sternocleidomastoid using the eccentric strength of the deeper anterior neck muscles to stabilize the weight of the head. Ustrasana can be an intense mobilization for the digestive system, especially the esophagus.

Breathing

In ustrasana, the thoracic structures are maintained in an inhalation position, and the abdominal wall is lengthened. This results in a decreased ability of the body to breathe "normally." The trick is to find support from the deeper musculature so that the more superficial efforts can quiet down. Then it's possible to notice an interesting relationship between the deepest layer of superficial neck muscles (scalenes) and the breath movement in the apex of the lungs, which are suspended from the inner scalene muscles.

Eka Pada Rajakapotasana

- *One-Legged Royal Pigeon Pose.*
- eh-KAH pah-DAH rah-JAH-cop-poh-TAHS-anna.
- *eka* = one; *pada* = foot, leg; *raja* = king, royal; *kapota* = dove, pigeon.

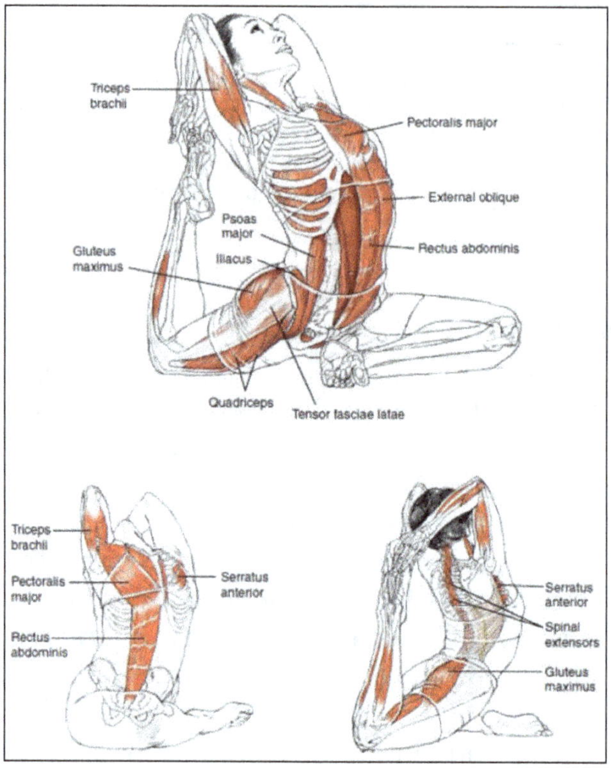

Asymmetrical kneeling backward-bending pose.

<table>
<tr><td colspan="6">Skeletal joint actions</td></tr>
<tr><td>Spine</td><td colspan="2">Upper limits
Front leg
Back leg</td><td colspan="3">Lower limbs</td></tr>
<tr><td>Extension</td><td colspan="2">Scapular upward rotation, abduction, and elevation; shoulder flexion, adduction, and external rotation; forearm supination; hand and finger flexion</td><td colspan="2">SI joint nutation, hip flexion and external rotation, knee flexion, ankle plantar flexion, foot supination</td><td>SI joint counter nutation; hip extension, internal rotation, and adduction; knee flexion; ankle plantar flexion</td></tr>
<tr><td colspan="6">Muscular joint actions</td></tr>
<tr><td colspan="6">Spine</td></tr>
<tr><td colspan="2">Concentric contraction</td><td colspan="4">Eccentric contraction</td></tr>
<tr><td colspan="2">To extend spine :
Spinal extensors</td><td colspan="2">To neutralize twist from position of back leg:
Internal oblique (front leg side) external oblique (back leg side)</td><td colspan="2">To prevent hyperextension at lumbar spine:
Psoas minor, abdominal muscles</td></tr>
<tr><td colspan="6">Upper limbs</td></tr>
</table>

Concentric contraction		
To abduct, upwardly rotate, and elevate scapula: Serratus anterior, upper trapezius To stabilize, flex and adduct shoulder joint: Rotator cuff, pectoralis major (upper fibres), anterior deltoid, biceps brachii (Short head)	To rotate forearm and grasp foot: Supinator and flexors of hand and fingers	
Lower limbs		
Front leg	Back leg	
Eccentric contraction	Concentric contraction	passively lengthening
To resist hip flexion: Hamstrings, piriformis, obturator internus, superior and inferior gemellus	To create hip extension and knee flexion: Hamstrings To create hip extension, internal rotation, and adduction: Adductor magnus	Iliacus, psoas major, rectus femoris

It is important not to collapse into this pose. The pelvic floor, hamstrings, and gluteals should act eccentrically to distribute the weight created by the force of gravity through the whole base of the pose rather than drop right into the hamstring attachment or knee joint.

As with all poses, and more so with complex ones, a wide variety of experiences are available, depending on each person's strength, balance, and range of motion. This pose is categorized as a kneeling pose because that is the starting position, but the base of support is not actually kneeling. This asana has a unique base of support: the back surface of the front leg and the front surface of the back leg. This same base, with the knee joints extended, would almost be hanumanasana. Even though the front leg is externally rotated, this pose still requires a great deal of length in muscles of external rotation such as the piriformis, obturator internus, and superior and inferior gemellus. This is because these muscles are also hip extensors and abductors, and the actions in the front leg are hip flexion and adduction—the more adducted the front leg is, the more sensation will probably be felt in those muscles.

When the knee is more extended in the front leg (toward 90 degrees of flexion), the rotation at the hip is greatly intensified. This action puts more pressure into the knee, especially if there is restriction in the hip joint, and the knee is much more vulnerable to twisting forces when at 90 degrees. The action in the feet and ankles can help to stabilize and protect the knee.

Eka Pada Rajakapotasana Variation

Folded Forward

This variation intensifies the actions in the hamstrings and other hip extensors (such as the piriformis) of the front leg because of deeper hip flexion and more body weight over the front leg. At the same time, it diminishes the actions in the back hip and in the spine.

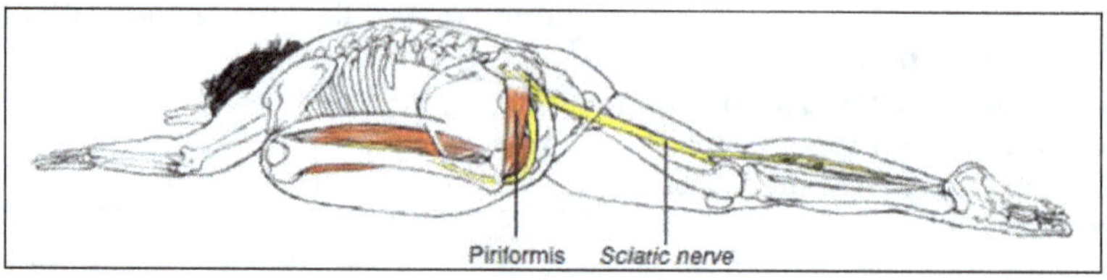

This position is frequently used to "stretch" the piriformis muscle and the sciatic nerve. When sciatic pain exists, however, it is not necessarily useful to stretch the sciatic nerve, and the piriformis is not always responsible for sciatic pain. It may indeed be true that doing this asana often helps relieve this pain, but it's more likely that the mobilization of the hips and pelvis and the effects on all the muscles of the lower body are responsible. The following illustrations show the relationship of the sciatic nerve to the piriformis muscle in:

- Neutral hip position.
- External rotation and abduction, which actually shorten the piriformis.
- Hip flexion, which begins the lengthening of the piriformis and other external rotators.
- Hip flexion combined with adduction, which puts the piriformis into maximal length, along with the sciatic nerve.

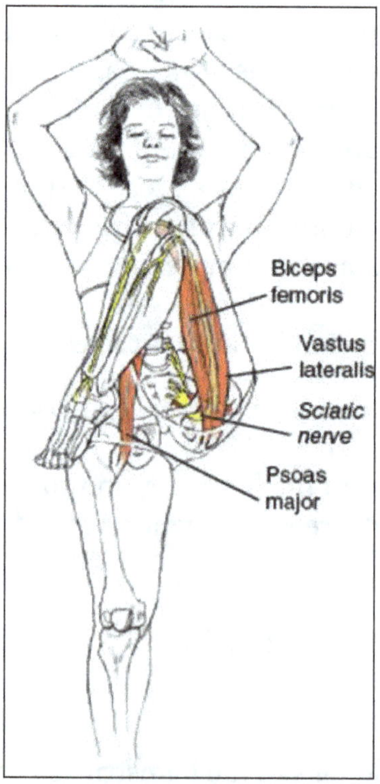

Folded-Forward Variation

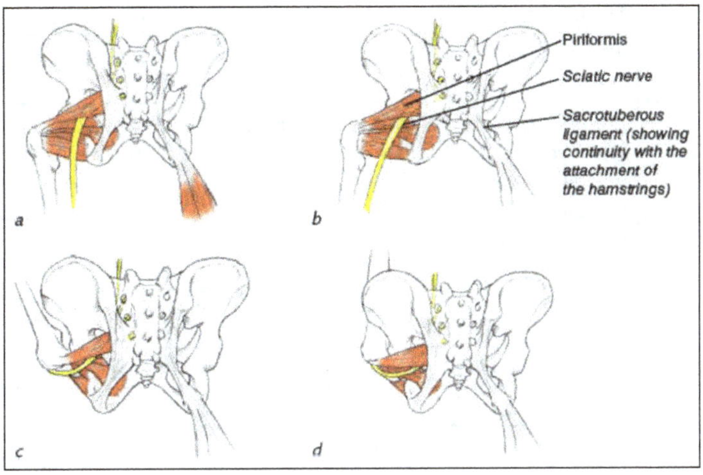

The hip joint, sciatic nerve, and piriformis muscle in four positions as they go into the folded-forward pigeon variation: *(a)* neutral; *(b)* externally rotated and abducted; *(c)* externally rotated, abducted, and flexed; and *(d)* externally rotated, flexed, and adducted.

Parighasana

- *Gate-Latch Pose.*
- par-ee-GOSS-anna.
- *parigha* = an iron bar used for locking a gate.

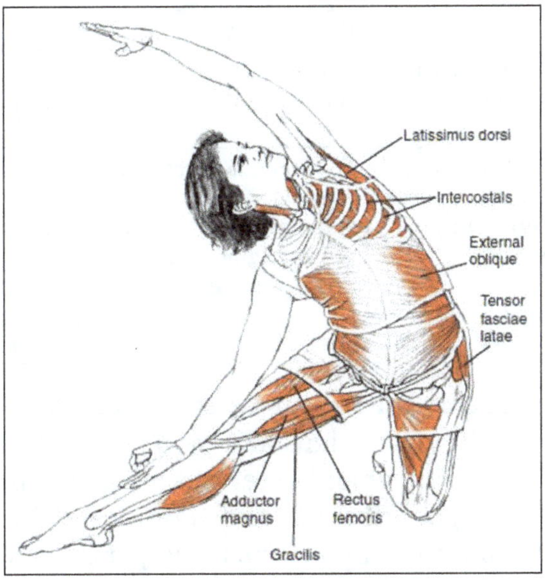

Asymmetrical kneeling side-bending pose.

<table>
<tr><td colspan="5">Skeletal joint actions</td></tr>
<tr><td rowspan="2">Spine</td><td colspan="2">Upper limits</td><td colspan="2">Lower limbs</td></tr>
<tr><td>Top arm</td><td>Lower arm</td><td>Kneeling leg</td><td>Extended leg</td></tr>
<tr><td>Lateral flex-ion, cervical rotation and extension</td><td>Scapular upward rotation and elevation, shoulder abduction, elbow extension</td><td>Shoulder abduction, forearm supination</td><td>Hip extension and adduction, knee flexion, ankle dorsiflexion</td><td>Hip flexion, external rotation and abduction; knee extension; ankle plantar flexion</td></tr>
<tr><td colspan="5">Muscular joint actions</td></tr>
<tr><td colspan="5">Spine</td></tr>
<tr><td colspan="2">Concentric contraction</td><td colspan="3">Eccentric contraction</td></tr>
<tr><td colspan="2">To orient torso to front:
Internal oblique (flexed leg side); external oblique (extended leg side)</td><td colspan="3">To resist falling into gravity:
External oblique, quadratus lumborum (flexed leg side)</td></tr>
<tr><td colspan="5">Upper limbs</td></tr>
<tr><td colspan="5">Upper arm</td></tr>
<tr><td colspan="2">Concentric contraction</td><td colspan="3">Eccentric contraction</td></tr>
<tr><td colspan="2">To upwardly rotate, abduct, and elevate scapula:
Serratus anterior
To stabilize shoulder joint:
Rotator cuff
To extend elbow:
Triceps brachii, anconeus</td><td colspan="3">To extend arm overhead without falling into gravity:
Teres major, latissimus dorsi</td></tr>
<tr><td colspan="5">Lower limbs</td></tr>
<tr><td colspan="2">Extended leg</td><td colspan="3">Kneeling leg</td></tr>
<tr><td>Concentric contraction</td><td>Eccentric contraction</td><td>Concentric contraction</td><td>Eccentric contraction</td><td>passively lengthening</td></tr>
<tr><td>To rotate and abduct leg: Sartorius, piriformis, superior and inferior gemellus, obturator internus</td><td>To keep from collapsing into hip: Hamstrings</td><td>To extend, adduct, and internally rotate hip: Hamstrings, adductor magnus, gluteus maximus</td><td>To resist hip extension and knee flexion: Rectus femoris To resist knee flexion: Articularis genu-vastii</td><td>Gluteus medius and minimus, tensor fasciae latae</td></tr>
</table>

Rotation is automatic with side bending in the spine because of both the shape of the articular facets in the vertebrae and the spiral pathways of the muscles. To keep the action pure lateral flexion, the upper and lower ribs need to counterrotate in relation to each other. In this case, the upper ribs rotate posteriorly and the lower ribs rotate anteriorly. To achieve this, the internal obliques on the upper side and the external obliques on the lower side are recruited.

Also, if tightness exists in the outside of the standing leg hip joint (in the tensor fasciae latae, gluteus medius, or gluteus minimus), then that hip will try to flex rather than stay purely adducted. The standing leg should maintain hip extension (via the adductor magnus and hamstrings) to prevent this. When there is tightness in the latissimus dorsi, lifting the arm overhead can push the rib cage forward (compressing the floating ribs and inhibiting breath in general) or pull the scapula downward even as the arm is lifting, potentially creating impingement of the biceps brachii tendon or supraspinatus at the acromion process.

Breathing

Which side of the diaphragm moves more in this pose—the upper, lengthened side or the lower, compressed side.

Simhasana

- *Lion Pose.*
- sim-HAHS-anna.
- *simha* = lion.

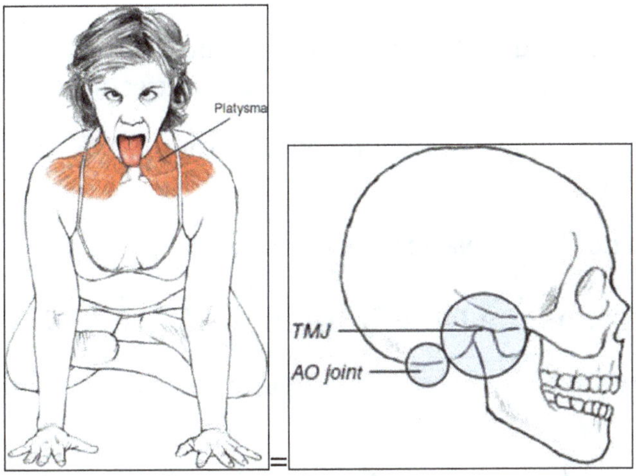

The temporomandibular joint (TMJ) represents the center of gravity of the skull, while the atlanto-occipital joint (AO joint) is its base of support.

Supine Poses

Supine Poses are poses done lying flat on our back with our face up. This means these positions are versatile, calming and accessible to all. Supine poses are great for every body type and all yogis, from those who have never tried Yoga before to advanced Yoga masters. Supine poses can be practiced by anyone and are also a great option for those who have difficulties standing for long periods of time. If someone is experiencing pain and pressure in the knees, for example, the laying position relieves the force of gravity against the joints and is therefore the perfect option to stay fit. There are various poses (asana) that can be practiced in a supine position that can be included in your Yoga practice or stand on their own as Yoga session.

Uttanpadasana (Double Leg Raise Pose)

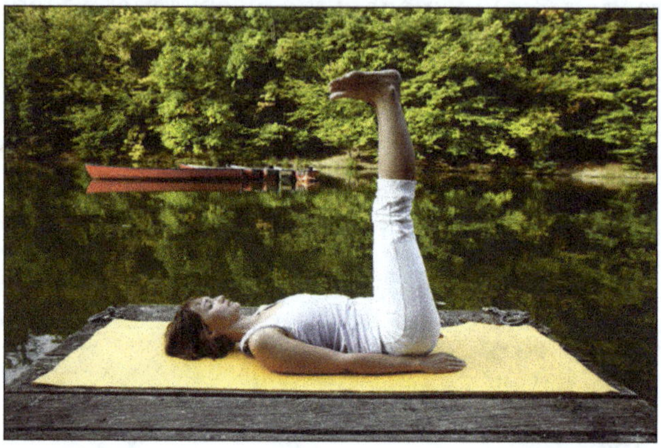

- Lie flat on your back with your ankles together and arms at your side with your palms facing down.
- Inhale as you extend and lengthen your spine. Imagine that a string is pulling the top of your head and your feet in opposite directions.
- Exhale as you lift your legs simultaneously. They can be raised up to a 45 degree angle or a 90 degree angle.
- Breathe and hold this pose for five breaths.

Supta Baddha Konasana (Reclining Bound Angle or Butterfly Pose)

- Begin by lying flat on our back with your arms outward and your palms facing upward.
- Bring the heels of your feet together as close to your pelvic area as you feel comfortable.
- Breathe, relax and let the power of gravity gently lower your knees toward the ground.

Pavanamuktasana (Wind Relieving Pose)

- Again, begin lying face up with your ankles together and inhale.
- With an exhale bend your legs and bring your knees up to your chest.

- Wrap your arms around your knees to carefully coax them to come closer to your chest.
- Bring your forehead onto or near to your knees. Be cautious not to strain your neck.

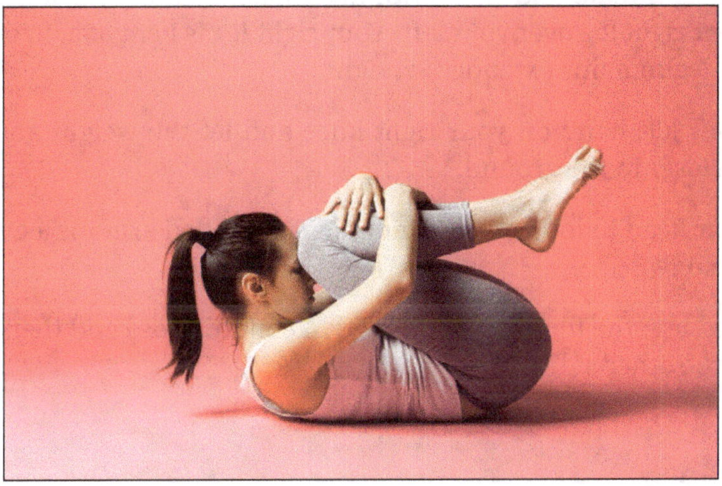

Setu Bandha Sarvangasana (Bridge Pose)

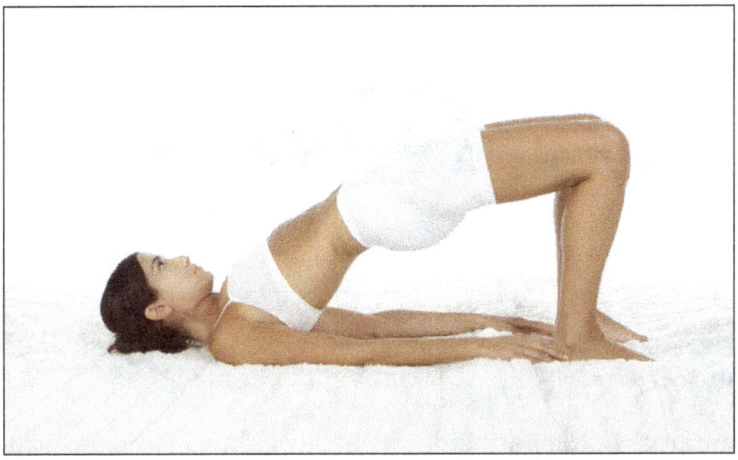

- As you lie on your back, bend your legs and place your feet directly under your knees.
- Slowly lift your hips upward toward the sky. You can use your arms to lift and support your lower back or extend them flat as you grab onto your ankles or hold your hands together.
- Use the muscles in your legs as support and bring your chest toward your chin. If you feel any pressure in your spine, use your hands to support yourself or hold the pose for less time, otherwise, remain here for five breaths.

Supta Matsyendrasana (Reclining Spinal Twist)

- Lie flat on your back with your arms extended straight out to resemble a cross.
- Take a deep inhale and then with an exhale, rotate your hips to the left and bring your right leg over your left. Your right leg is bent at a 90 degree angle and your left leg remains extended straight.
- Place your left hand on your right knee and let the weight and gravity gently bring it closer to the ground.
- Turn your head to look over at your right extended arm for a gentle and enjoyable spinal twist.
- Relax and breathe for as long as you'd like in this pose and then repeat the process for the other side.

Corpse Pose

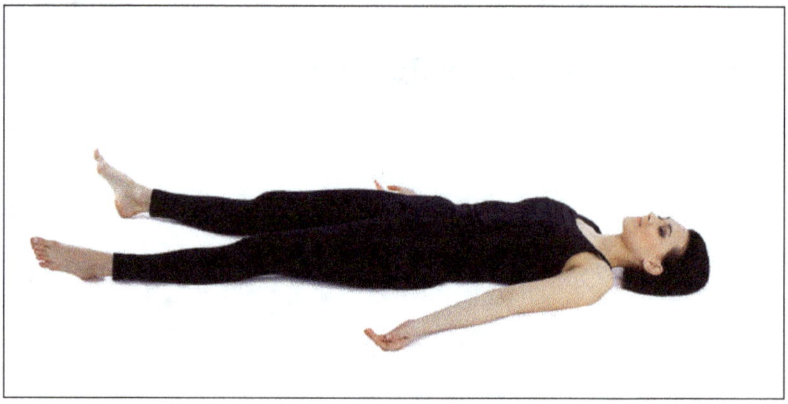

- Come to lie face up with your feet on the corners of your mat. Let them drop and point outward.
- Place your arms out at your side with your palms facing upward.
- Close your eyes and let your body relax and release all tension from every muscle, every organ, every pore, every molecule you get the point.
- Melt and enjoy for as long as you'd like. The longer the better.

Supine Poses have restorative qualities and can be practiced by anyone. Because they are so versatile, they are beneficial to those of all ages, gender and skill level. This specific sequence can even be practiced in the comfort of your own bed first thing in the morning or last thing before you go to sleep. Either way, they are a great way to start or end your day.

Prone Poses

Lying on your belly means prone position. Let your abdomen, chest and chin touch floor and look steadily at your front. Place hands near your thighs with fingers touching each other and palms flat on ground. Your feet should also touch each other with toes stretched backwards. Breathe slowly. This pose is called as vipareet shayan-sthiti.

1. Shalabhasana: Place your fists under your lower belly near groin. While inhaling raise both your legs up together from the waist without bending at knees. Do not lift head – let your chin be touching the floor. Hold on for some time (Locust/grasshopper pose). Bring your legs down slowly while exhaling and return back to original pose. Keeping fists under belly helps raising legs to a higher level. Raising single leg at a time is called as Ardha-shalabhasana.

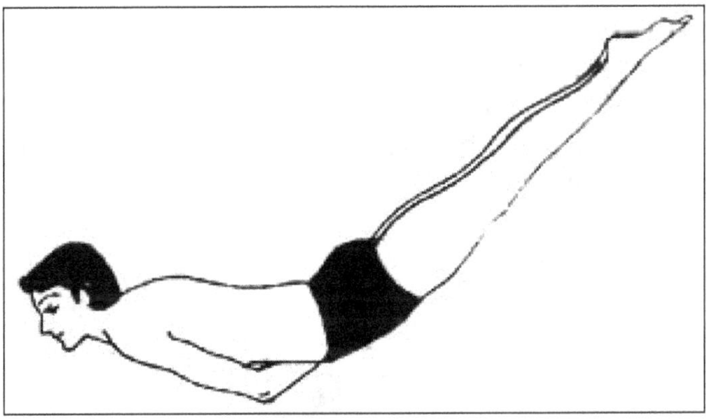

2. Bhujangasana: Place palms flat on floor at level of lower ribs. Stretch out both thumbs while keeping other fingers close together. Bend your hands so that elbows are directed upwards. Keep chin on floor. While inhaling raise your head, neck, shoulders and upper trunk (upto naval) one after other with help of your back muscles. Try to straighten your elbows without exerting much pressure on your hands. Do not strain your hip muscles. Take your neck as far back as possible and hold on for some time (cobra-pose). Come back to original position while exhaling to bring down abdomen, chest and chin sequentially. One can change position of hands as well as angle of elbows (vakra-hasta) to stretch spine at different levels.

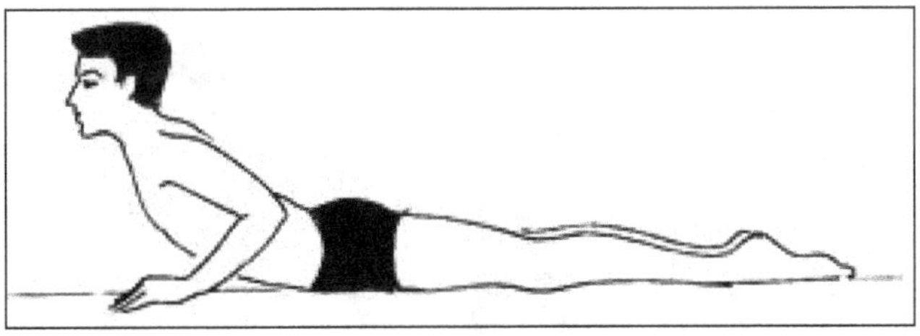

3. Sarpasana: Lie on your belly with elbows bent and palms flat on floor at the level of lower ribs. While inhaling raise your head, neck, chest and abdomen sequentially upto

the level of naval to make a backward curve. Hold on for some time (snake-pose) and while exhaling come back slowly to original position.

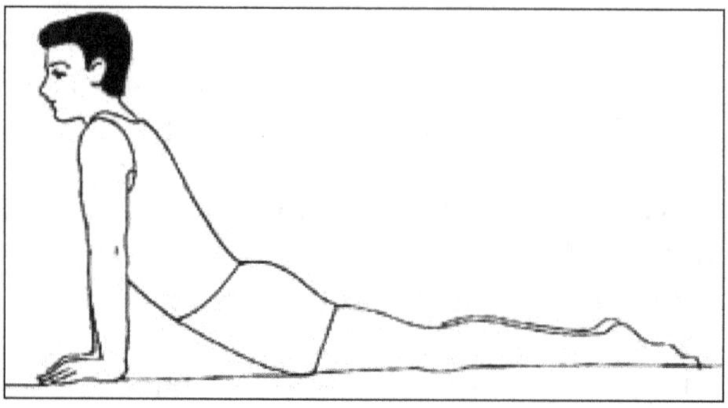

4. Naukasana: Lie on belly and place out-stretched hands in front of your head with palms touching each other (namaskar) and forehead touching the ground. While inhaling lift up your straightened hands and legs as much as (up to 450) possible. Your shoulders will now be near your ears. Let knees and feet touch each other. Do not bend knees. Hold for some time while balancing your body on your belly. While exhaling return back to original position.

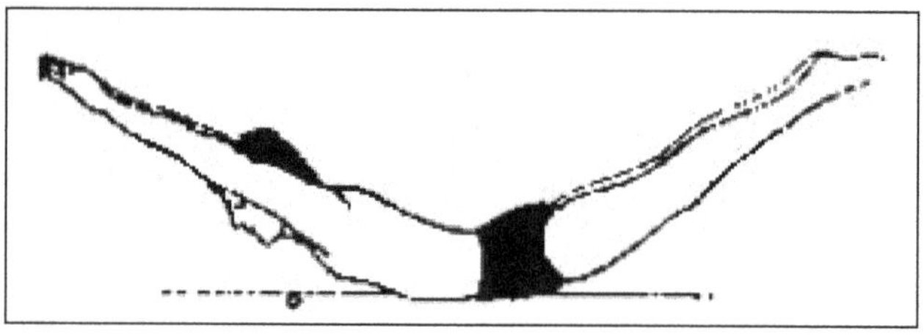

5. Marjarasana: Place your palms and knees on floor like a crawling child. Keep some distance between your hands as well as your feet so that your hands are beneath your shoulders and knees beneath hips. Lift up your neck while inhaling and press your lower back down. Hold on for some time, bring neck down and straighten up to original position. Now while exhaling contract your abdominal muscles and raise middle of your back straight up. Curl your head down to make an upward curve (cat-pose). Hold on for some time and return back to original position slowly. One can lift up a straightened hand and opposite leg, without bending at elbow and knee respectively, one after other in this position.

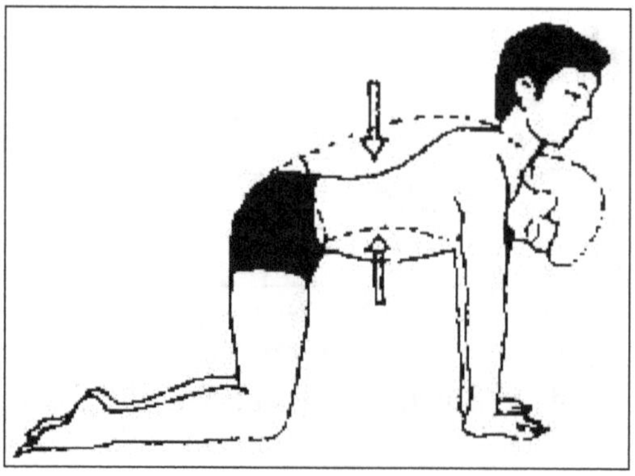

6. Dhanurasana: While lying on your belly bend both knees so that your heels reach buttocks. While inhaling bring both of your hands back and hold respective ankles. Now lift up your chest and thighs by pulling with hands. Raise your head too. Your entire body will now be stretched like a bow. Do not bend your elbows. Keeping knees touched together is ideal though difficult. Keep breathing quietly and hold on. While exhaling get your knees, shoulders and chin down to the ground. Release ankles and return to original position.

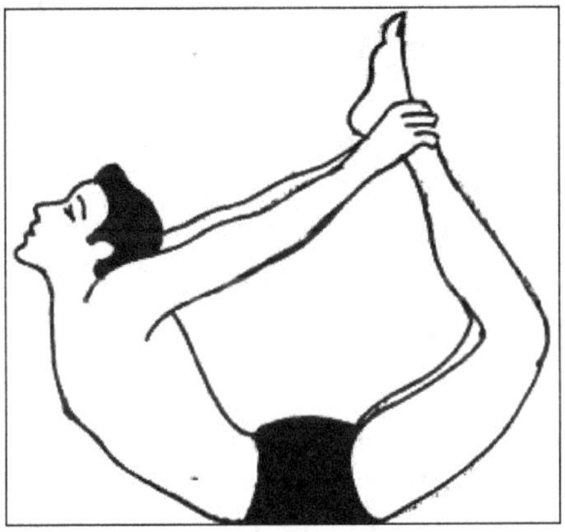

References

- Philosophy-286745: medicalnewstoday.com, Retrieved 10, August 2020
- Ground-your-home-practice-with-standing-poses1: yogainternational.com, Retrieved 04, May 2020
- Top-10-sitting-yoga-poses-asanas: rishikulyogshala.org, Retrieved 15, January 2020
- Yoga-anatomy: doctorlib.info, Retrieved 24, March 2020
- 6-simple-supine-yoga-poses: fitbodyhq.com, Retrieved 18, July 2020
- Asanas-in-prone-position: arthritis-india.com, Retrieved 29, April 2020

2

Branches of Yoga

Some of the prominent branches of yoga are hatha yoga, raja yoga, jnana yoga, karma yoga, bhakti yoga, tantra yoga and mantra yoga. Hatha yoga is the branch of yoga which is used as a form of physical exercise. This chapter closely examines these key branches of yoga to provide an extensive understanding of the subject.

Raja Yoga

Raja means King. A king acts with independence, self-confidence and assurance. Likewise, a Raja Yogi is autonomous, independent and fearless. Raja Yoga is the path of self-discipline and practice. Raja Yoga is also known as Ashtanga Yoga (Eight Steps of Yoga), because it is organised in eight parts:

- Yama: Self-control.
- Niyama: Discipline.
- Asana: Physical exercises.
- Pranayama: Breath exercises.
- Pratyahara: Withdrawal of the senses from external objects.
- Dharana: Concentration.
- Dhyana: Meditation.
- Samadhi: Complete Realisation.

The eight steps of Raja Yoga provide systematic instruction to attain inner peace, clarity, self-control and Realisation.

Yama – Self-Control

Consists of five principles:

- Ahimsa: Non-Violence: Ahimsa means not to cause pain or harm to any living being by thought, word or deed. Non-violence also means not to kill.

Consumption of meat requires the death of an animal. It is due to this principle that Yogis are Vegetarian. Animals have a keen instinct, which heightens their awareness of impending death. They sense when they are to be slaughtered and are in mortal fear. Fear and stress hormones are released throughout their body. These hormones remain in the flesh of the slaughtered animal and are eaten by unsuspecting people. Many apparently groundless fears, neuroses and psychoses have their origin in this food.

- Satya - Truthfulness: To always speak the truth is good and correct, but more important is how we convey the truth. We have the capacity to hurl truth at someone like a knife, but we are also capable of clothing that same truth in loving words. In order not to violate the principle of Ahimsa as mentioned above, we should heed the advice of Mahaprabhuji, who said: "Each of your words should fall like flowers from your lips".

  To be truthful also means not to hide your feelings, not to be evasive or make excuses. Perhaps for some time we can hide our true face from the eyes of others, but there is at least one person knows our inner truth - our own self. Our own consciousness is a witness.

- Asteya - Non-Stealing: Asteya means that you should never take anything that rightfully belongs to another. This means not only material objects, but also the stealing of mental property, to rob someone of an opportunity, hope or joy. The exploitation of nature and destruction of the environment also fall into this category.

- Brahmacharya - Pure Way of Life: Brahmacharya is often translated as sexual abstinence. But it actually consists of much more. Brahmacharya means that our thoughts should always be turned towards God. This doesn't imply that we should neglect our duties in this world. On the contrary, we should fulfil these responsibilities with great care, but always with the awareness: "I am not the doer, God alone is the doer".

- Aparigraha - Non-Accumulation of Possessions: We should not accumulate goods, but only acquire and use what we need to live. One who has many possessions, also has many worries. We are born without belongings and when we again depart from this world, we leave all behind. Nonaccumulation also means to grant other people their freedom - not to hold onto others. In letting go, we also free ourselves. Therefore, to give freedom means to also to be free one's self.

Niyama - Discipline

Consists of five principles:

- Shauca - Purity: Not only external purity, but more importantly, inner purity. Our clothing, our body, as well as our thoughts and feelings should be pure. The same holds true for the people we associate with. For our spiritual development it is of great benefit to keep good company of people who impart a good influence upon us, who are spiritual and support us with their wisdom.

- Santosh - Contentment: Contentment is the greatest wealth we are able to possess. The Indian poet Tulsidas, said: "You may possess mines of gold and precious stone, but inner discontent destroys all wealth". We can attain contentment only when we recognise that all worldly goods bring disappointment and that inner wealth provides more happiness than material possessions.
- Tapa - Self-Control, Self-Discipline: In life, when we encounter adversity and obstacles, we should never give up. Rather we should continue on our chosen path with firm determination. To continue to practice, with self-discipline, patience and perseverance - this is the key to success.
- Svadhyaya - Study of the Holy Scriptures: As Yoga aspirants we ought to acquaint ourselves with the traditional scriptures of Yoga philosophy, such as the Bhagavad Gita, the Upanishads, the Yoga Sutras of Patanjali, etc. These scriptures impart valuable knowledge and provide great assistance on our Yoga path.
- Ishvara Pranidhana - Devotion to God: Hand over all that you do to the Divine Self with pure devotion. God protects all who surrender with trust and faith.

Asana – Physical Exercises

Pranayama – Breath Exercises

In the process of controlling the body and breath, Raja Yogis also achieve control of the mind. This leads to an awakening of those inner powers which will continue to give guidance on the spiritual path.

Pratyahara – Withdrawal of the Senses

Yogis are in the position of being able to direct their mind and senses at will, either inward or outward. Just like a tortoise can withdraw its limbs and head under its shell and extend them out again. Once there is controlled Pratyahara there is gained an independence from external conditions. One can immediately withdraw the senses from external objects and also, when desired, use the senses consciously, with full awareness.

In the first stages of meditation we practice Pratyahara, keeping the body motionless, the eyes closed, the mind quiet and the attention directed inward. There are special techniques through which we can practice Pratyahara. One meditation exercise initially directs attention to external sounds, their nature, distance, etc. - simply observing the sound. Gradually awareness is withdrawn to one's "inner space" to the sounds within the body (heartbeat, blood circulation, etc.). It is only when one has mastered the step of Pratyahara that we can progress to concentration.

Dharana – Concentration

Dharana means to focus one's thoughts and feelings upon a single object. Usually we succeed with this for only a short time, then other thoughts come and distract us. We become aware of our lack of concentration after just a few minutes. Until we are capable of concentration on a thought or object for any length of time, in any situation, we still have not mastered Dharana. Candle meditation (Trataka), specific Asanas and Pranayamas, as well as the repetition of Mantra, greatly help in improving the ability to concentrate.

Dhyana – Meditation

All meditation techniques are only preliminary exercises for true meditation. One cannot learn to meditate, just as we cannot "learn" to sleep. Sleep just happens when our body becomes relaxed and quiet. Meditation happens when the mind is quiet. In meditation there is no imagination, because imagination arises from the intellect. We can compare the human brain to a powerful computer that has enormous storage capacity. All the data of the Universe may be stored there, but this "computer" is also limited. Our human brain can only reproduce what has been fed into it. But in meditation, we experience pure being. The moment the intellect is still and the individual ego ceases to exist, Divine light shines within the heart and we are one with it.

Samadhi – Complete Realisation

Samadhi is where the knower, knowledge and object of knowledge unite. The knower (i.e. the person practicing), knowledge (i.e. what is God) and the object of knowledge (i.e. God) become one. This means that one unites with the Divine consciousness. Those who attain Samadhi see a heavenly, radiant light, hear a heavenly sound and feel within themselves an infinite expanse. When Samadhi is attained, we are like a river that finally flows into the sea after a long and difficult journey. All obstacles are overcome and the river is, for all of time, united with the ocean. In the same way, a Yogi arrives at the end of the path and becomes one with the Supreme Consciousness. The Yogi's consciousness finds eternal quiet, peace and bliss - the Yogi is liberated. This experience cannot be conveyed in words, because:

only one who has tasted milk, knows how milk tastes;
only one who has felt pain, knows what is pain;
only one who has loved, knows what is love;
and so only one who has experienced Samadhi, knows what is Samadhi.

In this state all duality is dissolved. There is neither day or night, neither darkness or light, no qualities or colour. Everything is one in the Supreme Self. This union of the individual soul with the Cosmic soul is the goal of Yoga.

Hatha Yoga

The origins of hatha yoga have been traced back to the eleventh century a.d. The Sanskrit word ha means "sun" and tha means "moon," and thus hatha, or literally sun-moon yoga, strives to balance opposing parts of the physical body, the front and back, left and right, top and bottom. Some yoga masters (yogis) claim that hatha yoga was originally developed by enlightened teachers to help people survive during the Age of Kali, or the spiritual dark ages, in which Hindus believe we are now living.

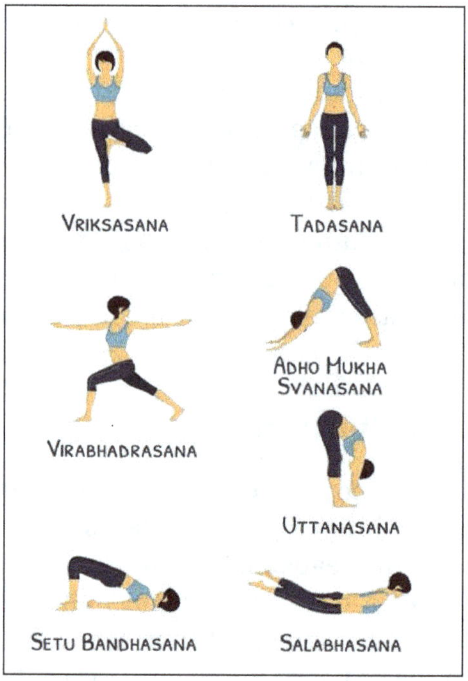

The original philosophers of yoga developed it as an eight-fold path to complete health. These eight steps include moral and ethical considerations (such as honesty, non-aggression, peacefulness, non-stealing, generosity, and sexual propriety), self-discipline (including purity, simplicity, devotion to God, and self-knowledge), posture, breath control, control of desires, concentration, meditation, and happiness. According to yogis, if these steps are followed diligently, a person can reach high levels of health and mental awareness.

As it has subsequently developed, hatha yoga has concentrated mainly on two of the eight paths, breathing and posture. Yogis believe breathing to be the most important metabolic function; we breathe roughly 23,000 times per day and use about 4,500 gallons of air, which increases during exercise. Thus, breathing is extremely important to health, and prana, or life-force, is found most abundantly in the air and in the breath. If we are breathing incorrectly, we are hampering our potential for optimal health. Pranayama, literally the "science of breathing" or "control of life force," is the yogic practice of breathing correctly and deeply.

In addition to breathing, hatha yoga utilizes asanas, or physical postures, to bring about flexibility, balance and strength in the body. Each of these postures has a definite form and precise steps for achieving the desired position and for exiting it. These postures, yogis maintain, have been scientifically developed to increase circulation and health in all parts of the body, from the muscular tissues to the glands and internal organs. Yogis claim that although hatha yoga can make the body as strong and fit as any exercise program, its real benefits come about because it is a system of maintenance and balance for the whole body.

Yoga was brought to America in the late 1800s, when Swami Vivekananda, an Indian yogi, presented a lecture on yoga in Chicago. Hatha yoga captured the imagination of the Western mind, because accomplished yogis could demonstrate incredible levels of fitness, flexibility, and control over their bodies and metabolism. Yoga has flourished in the West. Americans have brought to yoga their energy and zest for innovation, which troubles some Indian yogis and encourages others, as new variations and schools of yoga have developed. For instance, power yoga is a recent Americanized version of yoga which takes hatha yoga principles and speeds them up into an extremely rigorous aerobic workout, and many strict hatha yoga teachers oppose this sort of change to their philosophy. Other variations of hatha yoga in America now include Iyengar, Ashtanga, Kripalu, Integral, Viniyoga, Hidden Language, and Bikram yoga, to name a few.

A hatha yoga routine consists of a series of physical postures and breathing techniques. Routines can take anywhere from 20 minutes to two hours, depending on the needs and ability of the practitioner. Yoga should always be adapted to one's state of health; that is, a shorter and easier routine should be used when a person is fatigued. Yoga is ideally practiced at the same time every day, to encourage the discipline of the practice. It can be done at any time of day; some prefer it in the morning as a wake-up routine, while others like to wind down and de-stress with yoga at the end of the day.

Yoga asanas consist of three basic movements: backward bends, forward bends, and twisting movements. These postures are always balanced; a back bend should be followed with a forward bend, and a leftward movement should be followed by one to the right. Diaphragm breathing is important during the poses, where the breath begins at the bottom of the lungs. The stomach should move outward with the inhalation and relax inward during exhalation. The breath should be through the nose at all times during hatha asanas. Typically, one inhales during backward bends and exhales during forward bending movements.

The mental component in yoga is as important as the physical movements. Yoga is not a competitive sport, but a means to self-awareness and self-improvement. An attitude of attention, care, and non-criticism is important; limitations should be acknowledged and calmly improved. Patience is important, and yoga stretches should be slow and worked up to gradually. The body should be worked with, and never against, and a person should never overexert. A yoga stretch should be done only so far as proper form and alignment of the whole body can be maintained. Some yoga stretches can be uncomfortable for beginners, and part of yoga is learning to distinguish between sensations that are beneficial and those that can signal potential injury. A good rule is that positions should be stopped when there is sharp pain in the joints, muscles, or tendons.

Jnana Yoga

Jnana is Sanskrit for "knowledge or wisdom" and Jnana Yoga is the path of attaining knowledge of the true nature of reality through the practice of meditation, self-inquiry, and contemplation. Jnana Yoga can be defined as the "awareness of absolute consciousness," and is a comprehensive practice of self-study (Svadhyaya).

In Jnana yoga, the mind is used to inquire into its own nature and to transcend the mind's identification with its thoughts and ego. The fundamental goal of Jnana yoga is to become liberated from the illusionary world of maya (self-limiting thoughts and perceptions) and to achieve the union of the inner Self (Atman) with the oneness of all life (Brahman). This is achieved by steadfastly practicing the mental techniques of self-questioning, reflection and conscious illumination that are defined in the Four Pillars of Knowledge. Jnana Yoga utilizes a one-pointed meditation on a single question of self-inquiry to remove the veils of illusion created by your concepts, world views, and perceptions. This practice allows you to realize the temporary and illusionary nature of maya and to see the oneness of all things.

The Four Pillars of Knowledge (sadhana chatushtaya) are the prescribed steps toward achieving liberation in Jnana Yoga. These practices build upon each other and thus should be practiced in sequential order. Even if one does not have the goal of achieving liberation, practicing these techniques will cultivate spiritual insight and understanding as well as reduce one's suffering and dissatisfaction of life.

1. Viveka (discernment, discrimination) is a deliberate, continuous intellectual effort to distinguish between the real and the unreal, the permanent and the temporary, and the Self and not-Self.

2. Vairagya (dispassion, detachment) is cultivating non-attachment or indifference toward the temporal objects of worldly possessions and the ego-mind. "It is only when

the mind is absolutely free from the attachment of all sorts that true knowledge begins to dawn." – Swami Sivananda.

3. Shatsampat (six virtues) are six mental practices to stabilize the mind and emotions, and to further develop the ability to see beyond the illusions of maya.

- Shama (tranquility, calmness) is the ability to keep the mind peaceful, through moderating its reaction to external stimuli.
- Dama (restraint, control) is the strengthening of the mind to be able to resist the control of the senses, and the training of the senses to be used only as instruments of the mind.
- Uparati (withdrawal, renunciation) is the abandonment of all activities that are not one's Dharma (Duty). A simple lifestyle is followed that contains no worldly distractions from the spiritual path.
- Titiksha (endurance, forbearance) is the tolerance of external non-conducive situations that are commonly considered to produce suffering, especially in extreme opposite states (success and failure, hot and cold, pleasure and pain).
- Shraddha (faith, trust) is a sense of certainty and belief in one's guru (teacher), the scriptures and the yogic path.
- Samadhana (focus, concentration) is the complete one-pointedness of the mind.

4. Mumukshutva (longing, yearning) is an intense and passionate desire for achieving the liberation from suffering. In order to achieve liberation, one must be completely committed to the path, with such longing that all other desires fade away.

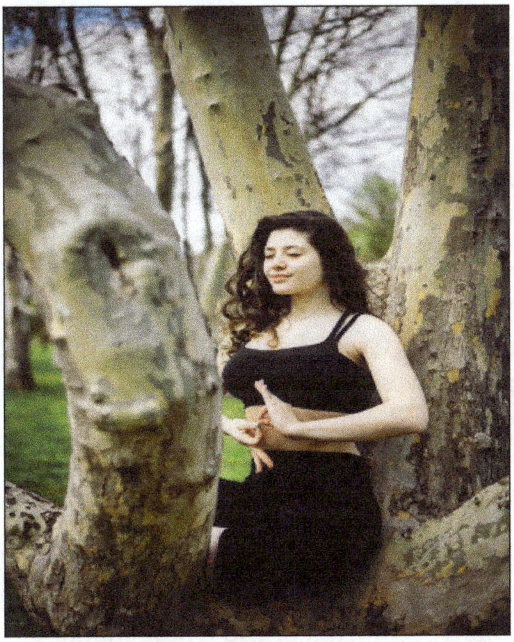

It can be difficult to grasp or comprehend the intellectual approach of jnana yoga, and since one can easily overemphasize intellectual attainment it is important to cultivate humility and compassion on this path. It is easy to become entangled in the constructs and thoughts of the mind and lose sight of the goal of jnana: to realize the divine oneness inherent in all beings.

It is recommended that one practice Hatha Yoga, Karma Yoga and Bhakti Yoga as prerequisites. These yogic practices will prepare and purify the body, mind, and heart for the rigors of Jnana Yoga.

Once you have attained some advancement in the other yogas, begin practicing the four pillars of knowledge. You do not need to feel you have mastered one pillar before moving on to the next, but do resist the temptation to progress forward before you are ready. This is considered an advanced practice and thus would be contraindicated for anyone with a history of mental disease or emotional instability. Working with a qualified teacher or guru is highly recommended to accurately assess your progress, offer individual instruction, and provide guidance for your progression.

Three Core Practices of Jnana Yoga

After one has studied and successfully practiced the four pillars, then you are considered ready to begin the Three core practices of Jnana Yoga. These Upanishadic teachings include sravana or "hearing," manana or "reflection," and nididhyasana or "meditation". These lead to Atma-Sakshatkara or direct realization.

- Sravana is the hearing or experiencing the sacred knowledge in the ancient Vedic texts of the Upanishad. Usually, a teacher or guru will guide the yogi through discussions on the philosophy of non-dualism. In this stage, the student should read and study the Upanishads and achieve a deep understanding of the concepts of Atman and Brahman and the philosophy of non-dualism.
- Manana is the thinking and reflecting on these teachings of non-duality. The student is expected to spend many hours thinking and contemplating on the various ideas of svadhyaya and sravana.
- Nididhyasana is the constant and profound meditation on the inner Self. This involves the meditation and reflection on the real meaning of the Maha-Vakyas, the primary mantras or "Great Sayings" of the Upanishads. Through the continuous focus on these seeds of wisdom, a yogi can obtain the union of thought and action, knowing and being.

The Upanishads Great Teachings

The Sanskrit word "Maha" can be translated as great or mighty, and the word Vakya translates as a sentence or saying. The Maha-Vakyas are the most revered and powerful sayings in the ancient Indian scriptures of the Upanishads. The regular contemplation and meditation of the Maha-Vakyas purifies our minds, promotes introspection and insight, and leads to transcendental states of awareness.

There are four main Maha-Vakyas but their contemplation leads one to the same realization. They present different points of view on how to see the indivisible oneness of all things. These four aphorisms also provide the answers to the classic questions of Jnana Yoga. "who am I?, What is my purpose? What is The nature of this reality?" These can all be answered by meditating on the Maha-Vakyas. The Four Maha-Vakyas are:

- Prajnanam Brahma: Brahman (Ultimate Reality) is supreme consciousness.
- Aham Brahmasmi: I am Brahman (The Supreme Self).
- Tat Tvam Asi: Thou art that.
- Ayam Atma Brahma: Atman (True Self) is Brahman (Ultimate Reality).

Jnana Bhumikas: The Seven Stages of Wisdom

Swami Sivananda describes seven stages that yogi will progress through while engaged in the practice of Jnana Yoga. Use this as a roadmap to gauge your progression and steer yourself skillfully towards your destination. You will need to overcome the challenges in each stage to move forward towards becoming one with the higher self.

- Subheccha (good desire): This beginning stage requires one to study the Sanskrit texts and be passionate about discovering the truth. One should strive towards non-attraction or indifference towards all sensual objects.
- Vicharana (Philosophical inquiry): The second stage involves questioning, contemplation and reflection on the principles of non-dualism.
- Tanumanasi (Subtlety of mind): This third stage assumes you have understood all the necessary knowledge. Tanu means thread, and in this step, The mind "becomes thin like a thread" as you let go of all external stimuli to focus all of your attention inwards.
- Sattvapatti (Attainment of Light): In the fourth stage, the world appears like a dream And your karma begins to dissolve. A yogi will view all things in the universe equally in this stage.
- Asamsakti (Inner Detachment): In this stage, you become detached and selfless and will experience deep states of bliss. One will feel no difference between waking and dream states.
- Padartha Bhavana (Spiritual Vision): In the sixth stage, you begin to see the truth and understand the nature of Brahman (Ultimate Reality).

- Turiya (Supreme Freedom): During the final stage, you are united in superconsciousness and attain Moksha.

Karma Yoga

Karma literally means "action". Action always comes with the consequence of the action. The law of karma is the law of action and reaction, illustrated by the well known saying "what we reap is what we sow", and also the law of retribution, which explains that "what we receive is the result of what we did in the past".

Nothing is by accident, merit, demerit, honor, or dishonor; any happening in our lives is the result of karma.The philosophy of karma is at the foundation of all oriental philosophical thought, Hindu and Buddhist. Understand how this law applies in life, helps us to spiritualize our life and progress.

Kinds of Karma

It is said that there are three kinds of karma: past karma, present karma and future karma. The three are inter-related and can be summed up thus, the present karma is the result of the past karmas, and is our reaction to the past, and will determine our future karmas. This body and mind are nothing but the result of past karma. These past karmic impressions have tendencies to reproduce themselves and determine the individual's circumstances and choices. These reactions to what has happened determine if they will learn the spiritual lesson or not.

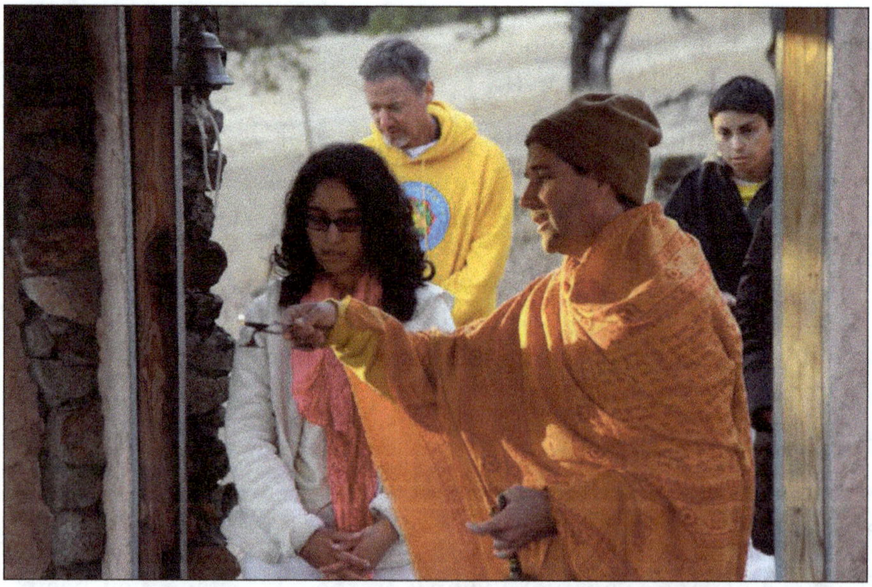

Swami Dharmananda waving arati lamp at Siva temple.

Karma is Neither Good Nor Bad

From the point of view of the Atman or soul, karma is that which binds us to the wheel of birth and death; the goal of the Yogi is to break through the chain of karma and release himself from all bondage caused by spiritual ignorance. This release from karma is gradual, as many lessons need to be learned and many experiences gathered for the individual to truly understand the Truth, which is the only thing that can set him free. Karma Yoga can be best defined as followed:

In this definition of Karma Yoga, there are 4 essential words: Duty, ego, attachment, and expectation of reward. To understand the principles of Karma Yoga, it is essential to understand these 4 principles.

The Four Principles of Karma Yoga

Duty

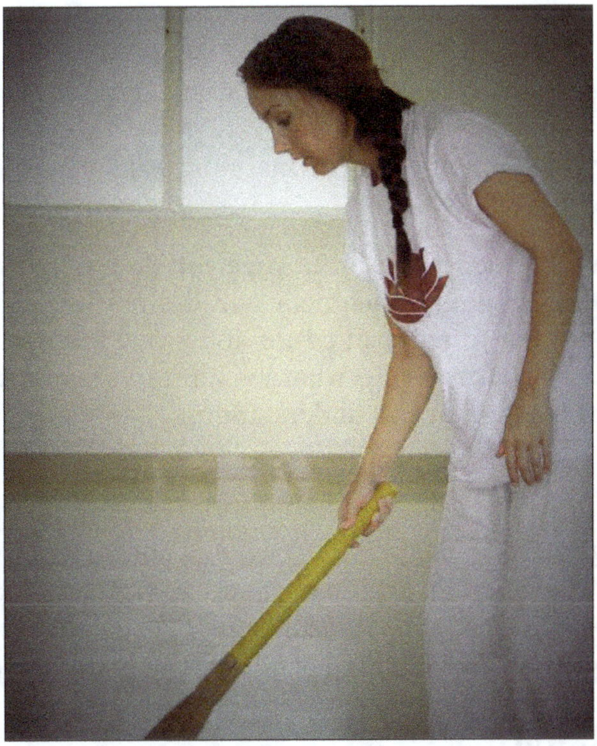

Everybody has duties in life. Some duties are given to you, you don't have a choice, for example, your duty as a citizen, as a member of society, as a son/daughter, as a brother/ sister, etc. Other duties you choose yourself, for example, your duty as an employer, as a husband/wife, as a friend, etc.

In Karma Yoga it is important to prioritize your duties; to know what is most important and which duty you should give more importance over other. It is important to realize that the highest duty you can have is the duty towards yourself. This means that you should first take care of yourself, do what is good for you and then only you can do what is good for others. For example, let's say you are ill and lying in bed. You should rest so you get better soon but late in the night, you get a call from a friend saying he feels lonely and he wants your company. Even though it is your duty as a friend to support your friend who needs company, at that time it is more important to take care of yourself and to get better before you can help your friend.

It is also important to fulfill your duty at your best. For example, if you are given a room to clean, you don't clean it very well because no one is watching or you think what you get paid for it is very less. Another example can be when your employer asks you to do something at work you have 2 options: you can do what he asks, nothing more, nothing less. You could have done it better and more detailed but because your working day was almost over you quickly finished the work and went home.

Ego

Ego is all the ideas you have about yourselves or others. It includes our likes, dislikes, desires, etc. With every action we do we tend to think about the consequences for ourselves; how does it affect ourselves, our image, etc. Karma Yoga is all about doing your duty without thinking about yourself. The main purpose of Karma Yoga is to control and eventually let go of your ego.

It is essential that in the practice of Karma yoga you do not involve your ego because only then you can do it without attachment and desire. Sometimes a person thinks he needs some ego in order to perform better and grow. But ego is like cancer which always keeps growing. It makes us see what we want to see and stops us from seeing reality. It controls our perception and understanding.

Attachment

Practicing Karma Yoga means doing your duty without attachment. Whether you like your duty or not, you still do it your best. You do your duty without any attachment for example if you are a teacher you don't teach one student better than because you like him more. You always perform your duty without any kind of attachment to the process or result.

Expectation of Reward

When we do something we rarely do it without expecting something back. For example, at the office, we do our work because we get a salary at the end of the month or for the praise or position. We take care of our partner or child, but we expect love and appreciation in return. When you do something without the expectation of reward, the outcome of your action doesn't affect if and how you do your duty. You do it because it is your duty, not because you get something out of it.

Misconception about Karma Yoga

There is some misconception about Karma Yoga, it is not:

- An exchange: Often people think if they offer their time and service in exchange for another service like a course or stay, it is karma yoga. If the action is done with intention of exchange, it is not Karma Yoga.
- Working for free: Working for free in name of spirituality or humanity is not Karma Yoga.
- Cheap labor: Working for cheap in name of Karma yoga is not Karma Yoga.
- Social service: Not all social service is Karma Yoga.

Remember, Karma Yoga is 'doing YOUR duty without ego, and attachment is Karma Yoga'. If your intention is anything else than doing a duty (natural or taken) without ego, it is not Karma Yoga.

How to Practice Karma Yoga

1. Right Attitude: It is not what you do that counts, it is the attitude while doing it that determines whether it is a job or Karma Yoga (i.e., a binding or a liberating job). Work is worship: Swami Sivananda advised that you should, "Give your hands to work and keep your mind fixed at the Lotus Feet of the Lord."

2. Right Motive: This is similar to right attitude; it is not what you do that counts but your real motive behind it. Your motive must be pure.

> Swami Sivananda says, "Man generally plans to get the fruits of his work before he starts any kind of work. The mind is so framed that it cannot think of any kind of work without remuneration or reward. A selfish man cannot do any service. He will weigh the work and the money in a balance. Selfless service is unknown to him."

Consider the example of two girls who were drowning. Two young men immediately jumped in to help them. One man jumped in so he could ask the girl to marry him. The other said only, "I have done my duty. God gave me an opportunity to serve and improve myself." The external action was the same, but the inner motive was different.

3. Do Your Duty (Swadharma): Often our specific duty in life is referred to as "Dharma", which means righteousness. Performance of duty frees the soul, and non-performance of duty keeps the soul in bondage. Perform your duty according to your caste and your stage in life, which are created by the Gunas or qualities born from a person's nature. The highest duty is to God, the In-dweller, to learn and to progress.

4. Do your best: Whatever you do, do your best. You will incur demerit if you do not give your best. If you know of a better way to serve then you must make use of it. You cannot hold back from fear of the effort required or from fear of criticism. Do not do work in a sloppy manner because no one is watching or because the work is not for you. Give your best effort. Try to do actions that can bring maximum good and minimum evil. Try at all times to accumulate merits. Do Karma Yoga increasingly often as this will accelerate your paying off of karmic debts. There is no time to lose. Swami Sivananda has said, "You can elevate others only if you have elevated yourself. A prisoner cannot liberate other prisoners."

5. Give up results: God is the Doer. You are not the Doer; you are only the Instrument. You do not know God's intentions or God's plans. God is the actor (i.e. the Self never acts). It is only the Gunas that are playing. The way to realize this Truth is to constantly work for work's sake and to let go of the outcome, good or bad. It is the desire for action that binds the individual. (I am the doer is wrong knowledge.) It is detachment from action (I am only the instrument is right knowledge) that will dissolve the Karmic seeds. Detachment from results also means detachment from the type of job itself. There are neither inferior nor superior jobs. Don't be attached to your job and be ready to give up your job when necessary. Note that Karma is always working. You will always be drawn to things that you need to learn. Staff smiling after baking cookies and giving to guests.

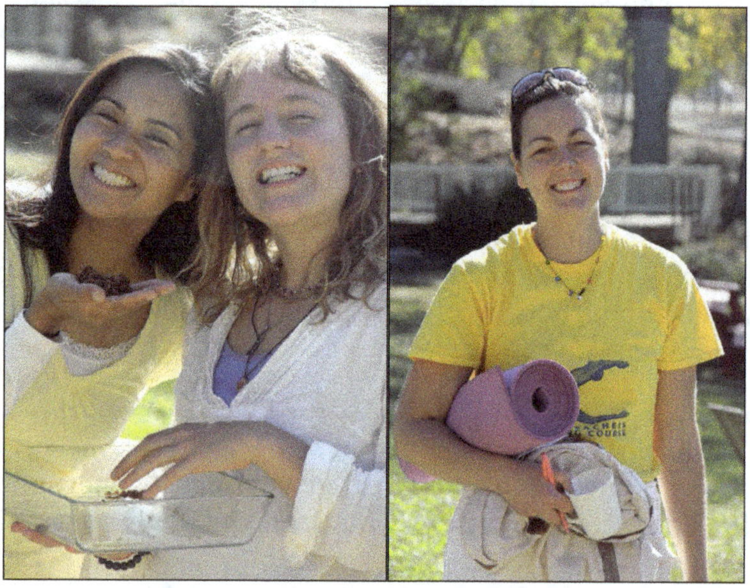

Student smiling with yoga mat under arm.

6. Serving God or the Self in All: Do unto others what you would like to have done to yourself. Love thy neighbor as thyself. Adapt, adjust, accommodate. Bear insult, bear injury. Unity in diversity. We are all parts of the same body. Practice humility in action. Beware of power, fame, name, praise, and censure.

7. Follow the Discipline of the Job: Every work experience has something to teach you. Try to do your best and the lessons of your work will be rich. Each job involves different requirements in terms of time, degree of concentration, skills or experience, emotional input, physical energy, and will.

8. Qualifications of a Karma Yogi: "A Karma Yogi should be free from lust, greed, anger, and egoism. He should try to remove these. He should be humble and free from hatred, jealousy, harshness, etc. A Karma Yogi should have an amiable, loving, and sociable nature. He should be able to move and mix with everybody without distinction of caste, creed, or color. He should have perfect adaptability, mercy, and cosmic love. He should be sympathetic and tolerant. He should be able to adjust himself to the habits and ways of others. He should always have a cool and balanced mind. He should have equal vision. He should rejoice in the welfare of others. He should lead a very simple life.

A Karma Yogi should have a sound, healthy, and strong physical body. He should do regular Pranayama, physical exercises, and Asanas in order to keep up a high standard of health. He should have the power of endurance." -Swami Sivananda.

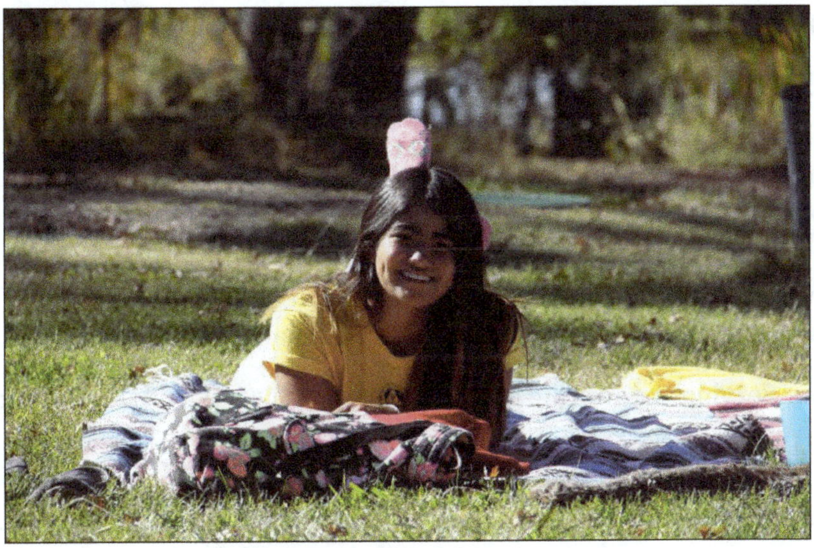

Student smiling lying down in grass.

What will the practice of Karma Yoga bring?

- You will develop and learn new skills.
- It will help personality growth, health, and fulfillment.
- It will thin out the ego and remove selfishness.
- You will achieve Purification of the heart.
- You will overcome the "likes and dislikes" of your mind.

- You will eliminate prejudices.
- You will feel oneness, unity and unbounded joy.
- You will become more loving, balanced, and sattvic.
- You will have a more flexible mind and a more tolerant attitude (less rigid).
- You will broaden your outlook on life.
- It allows you to spiritualize your activities.
- It will keep you focused on God throughout the day.

Bhakti Yoga

Bhakti as a form of union with the Infinite must be as old as human civilization. Formally it got recognized as a way of expressing love for the Infinite, or God, in Shvetashvatara Upanishad. Much later in Bhagavad Gita, it was considered a "marga" or a path to realizing the Ultimate Truth. It is elucidated further in Bhagwatam, as aphorisms made by Narada, in Narada Bhakti Sutra.

Flavors of Bhakti

The love towards God has various expressions or "bhava." They are:

- Shanta: Where the devotee does not express himself or herself too much, through singing or euphoric dancing but remains blissful and calm.
- Dasya: Serving the Infinite as his most faithful servant. Like Hanuman.
- Vatsalya: Loving God like one's child, like Yashoda.
- Sakhya: Loving the Infinite like a friend, Arjuna or Uddhava are shining examples.
- Madhurya or Kanta: This is the highest form of Bhakti, where God is one's lover, spouse, beloved. One achieves complete oneness with the beloved. Radha displayed this love, as did Meera or the Gopis of Vrindavan.

Bhakti Yoga is considered the easiest yogic path to master and the most direct method to experience the unity of mind, body, and spirit. While Hatha Yoga requires a strong and flexible body, Raja Yoga requires a disciplined and concentrated mind, and Jnana Yoga requires a keen intellect, the only requirement for Bhakti Yoga is an open, loving heart. But Bhakti Yoga complements other paths of yoga well, and it is said that jnana (knowledge or wisdom) will dawn by itself when you engage in the devotional practices of Bhakti Yoga.

This deeply spiritual practice draws heavily on the Hindu pantheon of deities. Each of these deities is seen as representing a humanized aspect of the single Godhead or Brahman – much the same way the Christian saints represent specific attributes and qualities of God. The use of Hindu deities in Bhakti Yoga can be a large obstacle for Western practitioners, especially for those with a deeply religious background. But the use of the Hindu deities is not required for this practice – in fact, finding your own object(s) of devotion will be all the more effective in achieving yoga (union) with the Divine.

There are nine main practices of Bhakti Yoga that can be practiced independently or together. Each of these limbs creates a specific bhava (feeling) that appeals to different inner constitutions of practitioners.

The Nine Limbs of Devotion

- Shravana: "Listening" to the ancient scriptures, especially potent if told by a saint or genuine bhakta.
- Kirtana: "Singing" devotional songs, usually practiced in a call-and-response group format.
- Smarana: "Remembering" the Divine by constantly meditating upon its name and form.
- Padasevana: "Service at the feet" of the Divine, which incorporates the practice of karma yoga (selfless service) with bhakti (devotion).
- Archana: The "ritual worship" of the Divine through practices such as puja (deity worship), and havan or homa (fire offering).
- Vandana: The "prostration" before the image of one's chosen image or representation of the Divine.
- Dasya: The "unquestioning" devotion of the Divine involving the cultivation of serving the will of God instead of one's own ego.
- Sakhya: The "friendship" and relationship established between the Divine and the devotee.
- Atmanivedana: The "self-offering" and complete surrender of the self to the Divine.

The most popular limb of Bhakti Yoga in the West is Kirtana (usually called Kirtan), with national and local Kirtan walas performing weekly in small to large cities. Bhakti Yoga can be practiced by itself or be integrated into other types of yoga or spiritual practices.

The Bhakti Sutras explain that bhakti yoga is both the means and the end: aparabhakti, or lower bhakti, is the way to cultivate and deepen devotion, and parabhakti, or higher bhakti, is union with the Divine—the ultimate goal.

The intrinsic nature of parabhakti is immortal bliss. On attaining it, one becomes free from suffering and completely satisfied, having no more desires. St. Anselm of Canterbury wrote: "I have found a joy that is full and more than full. For when heart and mind and soul and all are full of that joy, joy beyond measure will still remain." After the initial intoxication with bliss, one enjoys the delight of inner silence. In the depths of this silence, one realizes a complete unity with others, and comes to understand that we are all the same—there is no separation.

Lower bhakti, or aparabhakti, is the way we can prepare to receive the grace of higher bhakti. It is a way to channel and transform our powerful emotions into positive, creative expressions of love and devotion to God.

Three Stages of Aparabhakti

There are three stages that a devotee experiences on the path of aparabhakti: The honeymoon phase, the desert phase, and the state of surrender and grace.

The Honeymoon

Just as in human love, there is an initial phase of falling in love on the devotional path. This is a time when our relationship to our spiritual practice is new and fresh and filled with hope. We may try to find our way to God on our own, but usually we are drawn to a spiritual teacher to help guide us. In this stage, your teacher may shower you with love and attention, and in your meditation you may feel a new sense of stillness and peace. You may experience sensations of joy and light as you get an initial sweet glimpse of your inner Self, and you may find that you can't wait to sit in meditation.

The honeymoon stage usually involves some external forms of worship. You can create an altar, placing on it whatever has special meaning to you, such as a statue or a picture of your chosen deity, a candle, and/or something from nature. You may feel inspired to perform rituals with flowers, fruit, incense, and/or ghee lamps. Your teacher may give you a practice to do with a yantra.

The beauty of this path is that we can also offer whatever we feel to the Divine. There is no need to suppress any of our emotions. The sage Vivekananda said, "Only strive to intensify them and direct them to God."

Like the Sufi whirling dervishes who perform their dance as a dhikr, a remembrance of God, you can offer your love through dance, heart-opening asana, or some other form of movement. You can also express your intense longing to know God through writing devotional poetry or creating spiritual works of art. Or you can find inspiration and guidance by reading and sharing the spiritual writings of saints and sages, such as Kabir, Tagore, Rumi, and Mirabai.

Even if feelings of devotion don't sweep you off your feet, keep making effort. Everything you do—prayer, chanting, reading scriptures, meditation—is taking you a step closer to being aware of the Divinity residing in your inner heart.

Prayer is a simple but very effective way to connect with the Divine. Swami Rama said there are two kinds of prayer: ego-centered prayer and genuine prayer. In ego-centered prayer we approach God to petition for favors. Genuine prayer, on the other hand, comes from within.

In this inner sacred prayer, Swamiji said, we do not pray to an external divine principle, "but to the highest principle within ourselves—not for any external favors or gifts but rather only for the strength to face and resolve with serenity all of the many problems that fill our lives. Such prayers, which are completely selfless and pure, are always answered."

Genuine prayer includes gratitude. As Meister Eckhart said, "If the only prayer you say in your entire life is 'Thank you,' that would suffice." Upon waking up, before you get out of bed, give thanks for a new day and for all you have—even the simplest things, like clean water, sunlight, laughter.

Chanting is a powerful way to channel the emotions. Singing the praise and glory of the many names of the Divine lifts and purifies our spirits, whether we do it alone or with others. Gospel singers and kirtan artists electrify packed concert halls with sacred sound, opening minds and hearts to a higher reality.

Contemplation is an important companion practice to devotion. Knowledge helps us discriminate between that which is eternal and unchanging and that which is fleeting and impermanent. Without a solid philosophical foundation (jnana yoga), a devotee can get lost in mere emotionalism, with no clear direction and goal.

Start by studying an inspiring scripture, such as the Bhagavad Gita, the Bhakti Sutras, the Bible, or the Koran. You can reflect on just the verses alone, or choose a commentary and read a chapter a day. Contemplate how these teachings create a philosophical framework for viewing your life in a larger spiritual context, and how you can put the teachings into practice. You can also form a discussion group for deeper study.

Japa, or recitation of a mantra, creates a deep positive impression or groove in our unconscious mind. By strengthening the habit of saying our mantra daily, both in seated meditation and throughout our daily activities, our negative thought patterns start to weaken. Mantra gives our minds a one-pointed focus in our meditation, allowing us to deepen our connection to the Divine. To cultivate bhakti while you are doing your japa, you can rest your awareness at your heart center.

At the end of your practice, take time to sit quietly for a few moments or longer to enjoy the stillness. Open yourself to receiving divine love and wisdom. Practice releasing all your worries and concerns to the Divine and let yourself be nurtured and guided. Then, when you come out of your meditation, bring this spiritual awareness and sense of compassion to every activity in your daily life.

The Desert

None of us want the honeymoon phase to end, but if you are serious about your spiritual path, you will start to go deeper and find yourself in the desert phase, or what St. John of the Cross called "the dark night of the soul." This is where you do the real work, just as a seed has to grow its roots in the dark soil before it can blossom into the light.

The desert phase is a time of great effort and spiritual dryness, a time when you may doubt your faith and wonder why you are spending time sitting in meditation. It is a time of deep longing and despair. At this stage, a genuine teacher may push you away so that you are forced to go inward. At the same time, your inner teacher will be drawing you deep into the cave of your heart. In this phase, you are caught in a no-man's-land—neither fully outward nor fully inward.

This is a part of the journey that every seeker must pass through, often many times. The sage Ramakrishna used to say that we cry for everything except God. When we truly cry for God, he said, in the same way that a drowning man gasps for his next breath, then we will know God.

The Indian princess Mirabai left her kingdom and spent years wandering in search of Lord Krishna, writing songs of love and anguish: "Lost am I save for love of Thee. / None can know the depth of my despair, my moments of weariness. / Unless Thou stretchest forth Thy helping hand, / How can I reach the further shore?"

Separation can be more powerful than being with the one you love: when you are totally focused on the Beloved and your deep yearning for him, your mind and heart become purified with your tears of longing and your meditation becomes one-pointed. During this stage, try envisioning yourself being carried in the palm of God. Trust that the Divine One will bring you out of this dark night of separation, no matter how long it takes.

Faith

It took St. Teresa of Avila almost 20 years to make her breakthrough. Her problem, she wrote in her autobiography, was that she couldn't stop flirting with men. She finally came to realize that such attachments are actually the expression of an inner yearning for the Divine. When we take care of the deeper inner need, the outer attachments drop away by themselves. Swami Prabhavananda wrote that when we put the Divine first, it is like having a powerful magnet pulling us upward, away from the lesser pull of our lower urges.

It is important to remember that the inner work continues on the subtle level as long as we continue to make effort, even if we see no outer signs of progress. A student who once complained to his teacher that his mantra was not working was told, "How do you know?" "Nothing is happening," replied the student. "You do your work," the teacher said, "and let the mantra do its work. You can't see it but much is happening on the subtle level."

Acceptance

In the desert stage we need to allow the unspoken parts of ourselves to rise into conscious awareness. In recognizing and acknowledging these parts, we can learn how to cultivate compassion for ourselves and others. To do this, make a commitment to sit with whatever is troubling you—create a space for healing. Accept and offer your whole heart, both good and bad, without hiding from your emotional wounds, anger, fear, grief, shame, and unfulfilled longings and desires. In the Gnostic Gospel of Thomas, Jesus says: "If you bring forth what is within you, what you bring forth will save you. If you do not bring forth what is within you, what you do not bring forth will destroy you." We cannot run from our issues. Our issues are our spiritual practice.

Surrender and Grace

In the last stage of aparabhakti, worship is mainly internal. There comes a moment when you have exhausted all your efforts and realize you can do no more. In that moment, something in you will finally break open and let go. Then you become the final offering as your lower self-humbly surrenders to the higher Self within. In this act of internal surrender, you open yourself to receiving grace. The light of the Divine descends and manifests, and the lower self-rushes upward to embrace it. There is a sense of unutterable joy as waves of divine light flood your being, breaking through inner barriers, purifying your mind and heart.

Except in rare cases, we go in and out of these stages repeatedly. As we continue doing our practice we go through them at progressively deeper levels. Each time we pass through the darkness and emerge into the light, our capacity to receive grace further expands. And this, in turn, gives us the strength to go even deeper into our practice.

In the beginning stages of practice, there is usually a sense of ego-identification present in our acts of worship—"we" are making the effort and taking the credit for it. But at this stage, we surrender the fruits of our actions and let go of our identification as the doer. The more we are able to surrender, the more we can open ourselves to being a channel for Divine Light to manifest through our thoughts, speech, and action. This becomes true karma yoga, or selfless service.

The sages and scriptures extol the path of service and surrendering the fruits of our actions as the highest path. Krishna says in the Bhagavad Gita (12.12): "For concentration is better than mere practice, and meditation is better than concentration; but higher than meditation is surrender in love of the fruit of one's actions, for on surrender follows peace."

In this stage, we experience the sweetness of the honeymoon stage again, but now it is grounded in knowledge, because we have faced our inner darkness and have gained wisdom, strength, and compassion. This allows us to act in the world from a deeper place of inner stillness, with more clarity and love.

The three stages of aparabhakti are a preparation for the unfolding of parabhakti, higher love, when we are fully ready for it. Those who have attained parabhakti say that in this state, jnana yoga and bhakti yoga are one and the same—we go beyond all forms and merge into oneness with pure consciousness, the Absolute Reality.

Until that time, however, keep offering everything you do to the Divinity residing in your inner heart, whether it's your formal practice, your daily activities, or your relationships with others.

Tantra Yoga

The word Tantra means, "to weave or expand." The root of the word yoga is "yuj" which means, "union." Similar to some of the other 8 Forms of Yoga, Tantra Yoga blends elements of Raja, Bhakti, Karma, Kundalini, and Hatha practices. What distinguishes it from others is that it also weaves dynamics of other mystical practices as well such as: astrology, Ayurveda, crystals, and gemology to name a few. In utilizing these aspects, the Tantric practice aims to expand beyond perceived limitations of yogic philosophy and the asanas.

The comprehensive approach of Tantra Yoga incorporates conscious breathing practices, pranayama, and meditation, and may be practiced individually or in partnership with another. In both practices, the relationship between the micro (self) and the macro (others) is enhanced.

Vinyasa, as a moving meditation through postures, or asanas, also may be practiced partnering, as a blending of energies or as a sole practitioner. The aim is the same: to gain awareness of our strengths and weaknesses, the places where we resist union with ourselves and others, and cultivate the ability to consciously respond rather than unconsciously react to both our fears and desires. When that occurs, we reach a state of eternal bliss.

Five Tantra Yoga Practices

Peace Pose with Pranayam: Conscious Breathing

Begin in a cross-legged seated position, Sukhasana, or peace pose. Gaze down; if knees are higher than hip creases, sit on a yoga block or rolled up yoga mat to elevate the spine.

For solo practice, place hands in gyan mudra (also referred to as jnana mudra in some practices) with the tip of the index finger touching the tip of the thumb, extending out the other three fingers with the palms facing up and resting on knees or thighs. Gyan mudra, a yogic shape for the hands, is considered the prime mudra with many health and grounding benefits.

If practicing with a partner, sit back to back in peace pose, sukhasana. You'll want to align your spines: start by scooting your seats as close to one another as possible. Option to use prithvi mudra, tips of the ring fingers touching the tips of the thumbs, remaining three fingers outstretched but relaxed. This mudra creates a circuitry igniting the heart meridian, or line of energy that extends from the ring fingers, extends up through the arms and confluences at heart center in both the front and backside of the chest. Take five full breaths, focusing on smoothing out the length of the inhale to match the same length on the exhale.

Sun Salutations: Surya Namaskar

Start in mountain pose (tadasana/urdhva hastasana), standing at the top of your yoga mat. As an individual practice, you may like to practice facing a full-length mirror. In a partner practice, you could either practice facing one another or side by side. Bring palms to meet at heart center in anjali mudra (prayer gesture) or place one hand on your heart, and one on your partner's heart. Take five deep breaths.

Extend arms overhead, mountain pose, then bow forward, keeping your heart open and gaze forward, and release your head into a forward fold (uttanasana). Bring hands to shins or thighs and lengthen through your spine for a halfway lift (ardha uttanasana). Repeat three times.

Modified Side Plank/Partner Modified Side Plank Pose

Start in table pose, wrists aligned under shoulders, hands spread wide, and hips stacked over knees. For partner modified plank pose, you can lightly touch the crown of the head with one another while in table. Then extend your right shins behind you, toes curled under as you root right hand into the mat and open your chests towards one another.

For an individual practice, bring your left hand to rest over your heart as you stack your left shoulder over right so your heart is wide open. Your hips are also stacked creating a beautiful opening for what are considered our more vulnerable energetic centers: hips and hearts. In partner practice, connect left palms overhead. Enjoy five breaths. Return to table and then switch sides.

Partner Peace Pose: Entwined Sukhasana

Come into a loose, cross-legged position (typically the larger person in sukhasana first). Your partner then sits on your thighs and crosses their ankles behind your back. Touch your third eye centers (space between the eyebrows) as you both lengthen through your spines. You may choose to close your eyes or gaze lightly into each other's eyes as you inhale and exhale through the nose. Take five breaths, allowing a natural synchronicity of breath, with your palms resting on the backside of your partner's heart. Surrender to the intimate experience of both your and your partner's heartbeat.

Child's Pose (Balasana), Partner Child's Pose

Bring your knees wide to the edges of your mat, fold forward resting your forehead on the mat, arms extended overhead but resting on the mat. (If knees are sensitive, you can place the folded edges of a blanket behind your knees before folding forward or rest your seat and perhaps forehead on yoga blocks.) If shoulders allow, bring your palms to touch in prayer, symbolic of union with all aspects of yourself.

For partner child's pose, assume the same shape described above, with heads pointed towards one another. With arms outstretched, you can place your left palm down, and your palm up to connect with your partner's palms. It's said that our hands are an extension of our hearts. Envision your inhale emerging from your left palm, breathing in the essence of your partner, and exhaling through your right palm, sharing your essence with your partner.

For a more advanced practice, presuming both partners have healthy knees and spines, you may like to have one partner (typically the larger partner) stay in child's pose, and the other, sit facing the opposite direction, on the low back of the partner in child's pose. Slowly, keeping weight in your feet, begin to lower down, using the support of hands on the mat alongside the bottom partner's hips. Eventually, lower your spine to align with the partner in child's pose, and relax arms alongside, or extend your arms overhead, sliding palms underneath your partner's palms. Stay in close communication with your partner in child's pose to ensure that each of the actions feels safe and available in their body.

Expand your Capacity for Intimacy

If you're practicing Tantra Yoga on your own or with a partner, you're expanding your capacity for intimacy and union. With practice, we're able to get up close and intimate with the beliefs and behaviors that hold us back from the intimacy we desire. In addition, Tantric techniques are provided to evolve beyond these barriers so that each and every one of us may thrive and prosper. The benefits of tantra yoga are:

- Awaken Your Spiritual Side.
- Increase Flexibility.
- Enhance Your Sex Life.

- Deepen Your Bond with a Partner.
- Promote Health and Wellbeing.
- Relieve Stress.
- Awaken Kundalini energy.
- It is the blend of eight form yoga.
- Provide Mental Clarity.

Mantra Yoga

Mantra Yoga has its origin in Vedic Sciences and also in Tantra, infact all the verses in Vedas are called mantras, it is said that any person who can chant or sing Vedas can achieve the ultimate salvation or union with supreme consciousness only by chanting the mantras, which is the aim Mantra Yoga.

Mantra Yoga or Japa Yoga

MAN + TRA - Mantra is a Sanskrit word made up of two verbs, Man & Tra which in sanskrit "Mananat Trayate", just by chanting one can save himself in the universe that is achieve the ultimate in this material world.

Easiest but safest way to pratyahara or sense withdrawal: Mantra Yoga is a easiest way to achieve difficult state of Pratyahara, that is Internalizing the sense oriented mind from external world and focus on inner consciousness.

1. Achieving samadhi (through rotation of consciousness): When you chant Mantra, you are repeating the particular combination of words, which is rotating your awareness around the combination, this particular repetitive action leads to awakening powerful inner force, if controlled properly this can lead to ultimate salvation or union with super consciousness. One can compare example of concentrated sun beams in Convex lens, the rays/beams can burn a paper if lens is used, similarly the consciousness/awareness can be made concentrated and powerful by repetitive chanting of Mantra.

2. Mantra - grouping of sound vibrations (affect mental & psychological plane): Mantra is nothing but a combination or grouping of various alphabets/"Akshar" as is called in Sanskrit. The combined effect of sound vibrations on physical plane can be observed, specially on brain, or on EEG (Electro Encephala Graph) one can see the brain wave emission patterns affected with Omkar chanting, Gayatri Mantra chanting. A alpha activity in brain can be seen during the Mantra Chanting Also Mantra affects subconscious mind, it has different impressions on sub conscious, thinking patterns are

affected, negative impressions can be removed from subconscious such as fear, anger, jealousy etc. also positive impressions can be programmed in the subconscious. Practice of Mantra increases concentration, memory, logical thinking. Mantra Chanting has soothing effect on Nervous System, helps relax the muscles, can be effectively used to reduce stress and its effects.

Requirements of Mantra Yoga

Guru mantra or in dreams: In Sanskrit texts millions of mantras are there, so the question is how and what to choose? Guru is the best judge of the disciple, he knows his disciples inside out. So guru can select a best suited mantra which will help and evolve the disciple. Sometimes people see the Mantra in their dreams. But this is very rare phenomena.

Universal mantra om - If one can't meet his guru, he can select the universal mantra mantra - nature of individual - The selection of mantras is based on the nature of individual, his mind, physique and spiritual stage of development. For example:

- Gayatri Mantra relate to sympathetic nervous system, so if a person is aggressive in nature and starts chanting Gayatri, he may start getting angry early as Gayatri Mantra triggers Sympathetic activities.
- Mahamrutyunjay - parasympathetic nervous system.
- Pouranic mantra (Om namah shivay, Hare ram hare krishna, Om namo narayan).

Generally Mantras can be classified in 2 categories:

- Tantric Mantras: This mantras has origin in Tantras, thousands of different mantras exists and they can be practiced for specific purposes, such as achieving wealth, health, success, curing specific diseases, longevity or even for doing bad to someone. But this mantras to be learnt from Guru and has lot of restrictions. The effects are also fast for these mantras. These mantras are difficult to learn.
- Pouranic Mantras: This are relatively simple and can be practiced by anyone, they are easy to learn and helps purify emotions of human mind. These mantras are safe, slowly the practice of these mantras leads to ultimate salavation.

Total faith in Mantra - One must have complete faith in the mantra, without faith even the medicine is useless, so absolute belief is necessary before practicing mantras.

- Yantra: Psychic shape of mantra, an impression of mantra in the subconscious mind has great significance, one can focus on these during the chanting of the mantra and increase the effects of mantra or achieve the results faster. Popular Shree Yantra, Laxmi Yantra are also associated with related Mantras, it is said that if one focuses on the yantras, he still can get the same benefits as that of chanting the mantra.

State of Consciousness in Mantra

- Relaxed and concentrated state of mind: Due to withdrawal from the material thoughts, distractions, focusing of mind only on Mantra, mind is relaxed and becomes concentrated. Research shows the presence of alpha wave/rhythm of brain.
- Rotation of consciousness around Mantra: Awareness is revolved round the mantra, its pronunciation, yantra (psychic shape) and its meaning, which builds up psychic energy which can then be used for spiritual purposes.
- "Sakshi Bhav": Attitude of unconcerned observer, this particular attitude is very important as it allows bypassing or witnessing disturbances arising in the conscious & sub conscious mind. Thoughts are generally very difficult to negotiate, this approach of "Sakshi Bhav" allows to overcome this problem.
- Lost awareness of outside world: When practitioner goes deep in to the meditation states while chanting mantra, there is absolutely no awareness about happenings in surrounding environment.
- Only Mantra awareness remains: Even there is no self, the mantra & its awareness is present when practitioner reaches higher states.

Methods of Chanting Mantra

- Baikhari (Audible): By chanting a loud which can be heard easily is called "Baikhari" Chanting. Advantages of Baikhari Chanting:
    - Removes thoughts.
    - Easy conceptualization of thoughts.
    - Makes meditation easy.
- Upanshu (whispering): Chanting of mantra in low voice, or just whispering so that only practitioner can understand is called "Upanshu" Chanting. Advantages of "Upanshu":
    - Long duration chanting (8 to 10 hours).
    - Purposeful Mantra repetition (example: for wealth, health, land acquisition, happiness etc.).
    - Destiny Errors can be corrected with this type of chanting.
- Manasik (Mental): Without chanting a loud or whispering, mantra is repeated in mind, this type of mantra chanting is difficult and can be learnt only with practice. Advantages of Mental Chanting:
    - Subtle form of chanting.

- Commonly used by advance practitioners.
- Leads to higher states of awareness.

Effects of Mantra

On Personal Level:

- Mantra impacts on mental & psychological plane in a positive way.
- Stirs up emotions (desires, fears, jealousy from subconscious mind to conscious level as thoughts.) for removing negative tendencies of mind and re programming the thinking process.
- Creates potential energy reservoir.

On Surroundings:

- Deeper, subtle & astral spheres.
- Impacts on macro cosmos & micro cosmos.
- Purification of collective conscious mind. Ex: feel good factor with swamis & yogis.

How to Practice

One should have a Mala or Rosary consisting of 108 beads as is significant in all Tantra & Veda Texts. Repeat Mala for 2 to 3 times daily (increase to even 8 to 10 hours) or Chant Mantra for at least 11 times. Time of Practice - Morning or evening time.

Pranayama during Mantra - Breath and Mantra (So ham with breath) One can chant the Mantra while exhaling or inhaling or both. While breathing a subtle sound of "So" can be heard and while exhaling "Ham", which is a repetition of Mantra "So Ham?"

Concentration on object of faith - One should concentrate on following objects during the practice:

- God.
- Yantra - psychic symbol of mantra.
- Purpose of Mantra on Paper.
- Stars in sky.

Rules of Mantra Chanting

Selection - Name of GOD, Guru Mantra, in dreams, OM as universal mantra.

Mala or rosary - 108 beads + 1 Sumeru (offset bead).

Types of mala:

- Rudraksha Mala - This is generally used for Mantra from Vedas, where long duration Mantra Chanting is practiced.
- Tulsi - Guru mantra.
- Crystal - Purpose of different malas:
    - Use middle finger and thumb only.
    - Practice Mantra in meditative pose.
    - Mala or rosary not visible to others.
    - Japa Mala should not be worn.
    - Do not cross sumeru (offset bead).

References

- Raja-yoga, the-four-paths-of-yoga: yogaindailylife.org, Retrieved 28, June 2020
- Ashtanga-Yoga-chart: mysorehathayoga.com, Retrieved 02, March 2020
- Four-principles-of-karma-yoga: arhantayoga.org, Retrieved 14, January 2020
- Bhakti-yoga-what-bhakti-yoga: artofliving.org, Retrieved 19, August 2020
- A-seekers-guide-to-bhakti-yoga: yogainternational.com, Retrieved 06, April 2020
- Tantra-yoga-guide-practitioners: gaia.com, Retrieved 01, July 2020
- What-is-tantra-yoga: mantrayogameditation.org, Retrieved 14, February 2020

3

Yoga Physiology and Doctrine

The human body within the domain of yoga is considered to be composed of five koshas, or sheaths. It also comprises energy channels which can be influenced and stimulated through yoga practice. The topics elaborated in this chapter will help in gaining a better perspective about the different aspects of human body in yoga such as kosha, chakra and nadi.

Yoga Physiology

Yoga physiology are the descriptions of the human body, its layers, and the energy channels running through it used in various yoga systems.

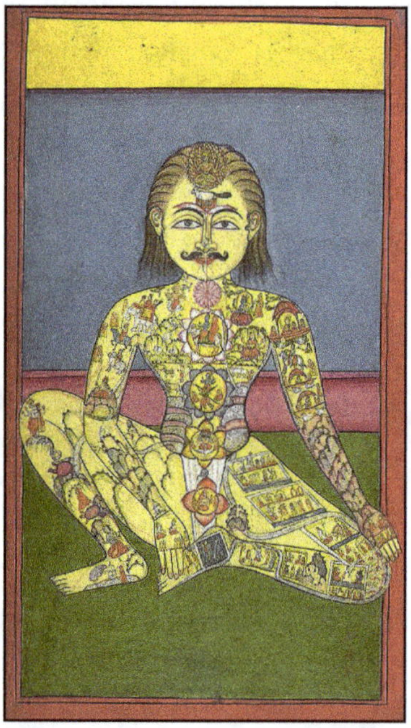

From an 1899 yoga manuscript in the Braj Bhasa language.

Yoga

DIALOGUE BETWEEN SHIVA AND PARVATHI (OLD HISTORY): According to a story in the puranas, Lord Shiva was instructing parvati into the secret sadhanas of yoga while standing on the seashore. A large fish overheard all that said and from this fish, all knowing Matsyendranath was born. Hence his name Matsya - Indra or 'Lord of fish'. There are also many stories concerning the birth of Goraknath. It is said that when Matsyendranath was begging for food as a parivrajaka, he met a woman who lamented to him her woe of not having a son. Matsyendranath gave her some siddha vibhooti and told her that if she eats it, she would obtain a son. The woman did not eat that substance but cast it upon a pile of cowdung. Twelve years later, when Matsyendranath was passing through the same village, he called her to see the child. The woman told the yogi what she had done and he asked to be taken to the spot where she had thrown the vibhooti. He called the name 'Gorkhnath' and immediately a radiant twelve-year-old lad emerged from the pile of cow dung. Gorkhnath became the dutiful disciple of Matsyendranath and later became an expounder of hatha yoga and the founder of the Nath sect. He was an accomplished guru credited with the performance of many miracles. Gorkhantha, who was probably the guru of Swatmarama, belonged to a very popular yoga sect called the Nath panth. Nath is a general term meaning 'master'. Members of these are Kanphata yogis. Kanphata means 'split-eared' and refers to the yogis' unique practice of having the cartilage of the ears pierced for the insertion of huge earrings.

Yoga are the physical, mental, and spiritual practices or disciplines which aim at transforming body and mind. The term denotes a variety of schools, practices and goals in Hinduism, Buddhism (including Vajrayana and Tibetan Buddhism) and Jainism, the best-known being Hatha yoga and Raja yoga. The term yoga is derived from the literal meaning of Sanskrit root "yuj" which means "to unite" ,Template:Monier Monier-Williams. A Sanskrit-English Dictionary: ...with Special Reference to Greek, Latin, Gothic, German, Anglo-saxon.. Clarendon. p. 804.

The origins of Yoga may date back to pre-vedic Indian traditions. The earliest accounts of yoga-practices are to be found in the Buddhist Nikayas. Parallel developments were recorded around 400 CE in the *Yoga Sutras of Patanjali*, which combines pre–philosophical speculations and diverse ascetic practices of the first millennium BCE with Samkhya-philosophy. Hatha yoga emerged from tantra by the turn of the first millennium.

Three Bodies and Five Sheets

According to the Doctrine of the Three bodies in the Vedanta and Yoga, the human being is composed of three Sariras or "bodies". They are often equated with the five koshas (sheets), described in the Taittiriya Upanishad which cover the Atman or "Self". They are:

1. Sthula sarira, the Gross body, composed of the *Annamaya Kosha*.
2. Suksma sarira, the Subtle body, composed of:
    1. *Pranamaya Kosha* (Vital breath or Energy),
    2. *Manomaya Kosha* (Mind),
    3. *Vijnanamaya Kosha* (Intellect).
3. Karana sarira, the Causal body, composed of the *Anandamaya Kosha* (Bliss).

Karana sarira is the cause of *Sthula sarira* and *Suksma sarira*.

Chakras

Chakras are energy centers or vortices in the subtle body. They are located at the physical counterparts of the major plexuses of arteries, veins and nerves. Chakras are part of the subtle body, not the physical body, and as such are the meeting points of the subtle (non-physical) energy channels, called nadiis. Nadiis are channels in the subtle body through which the life force (prana), or vital energy moves. Various scriptural texts and teachings present a different number of chakras. There are many chakras in the subtle human body according to the tantric texts, but there are 7 chakras that are considered to be the most important ones.

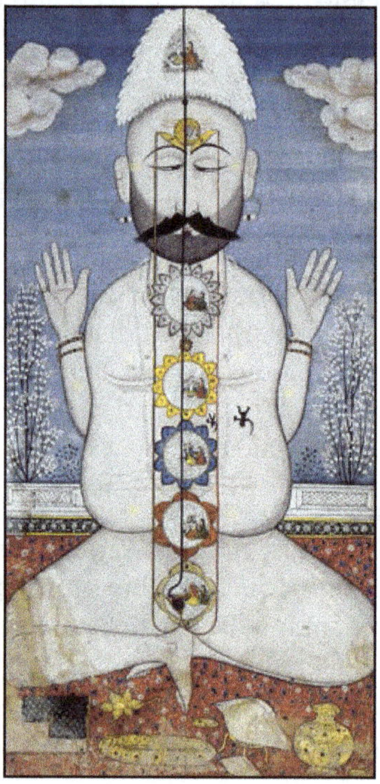

Yogin with six chakras, India, Punjab Hills, Kangra, late 18th century.

Their name derives from the Sanskrit word for "wheel" or "turning", but in the yogic context a better translation of the word is 'vortex or whirlpool'.

Nadi

Nāḍi (tube, pipe") are the channels through which, in traditional Indian medicine and spiritual science, the energies of the subtle body are said to flow. They connect at special points of intensity called chakras.

The word "nadi" is pronounced as "naRdi", with R+d loosely pronounced together (the effort is made by the tip of the tongue; it curls up, pointing backwards, then springs forward to lie flat). In normal biological reference, a *nadi* can be translated into "nerve" in English. However, in yogic, and specifically in Kundalini yoga reference, a nadi can be thought of as a channel (not an anatomical structure). In regard to Kundalini yoga, there are three of these nadis: Ida, *pingala*, and *sushumna*. Ida (spoken "iRda") lies to the left of the spine, whereas *pingala* is to the right side of the spine, mirroring the ida. *Sushumna* runs along the spinal cord in the center, through the seven chakras – Mooladhaar at the base, and Sahasrar at the top (or crown) of the head. It is at the base of this sushumna where the Kundalini lies coiled in three and a half coils, in a dormant or sleeping state.

Three Bodies Doctrine

According to Sarira Traya, the Doctrine of the Three bodies in Hinduism, the human being is composed of three sariras or "bodies" emanating from Brahman by avidya, "ignorance" or "nescience". They are often equated with the five koshas (sheaths), which cover the atman. The *Three Bodies Doctrine* is an essential doctrine in Indian philosophy and religion, especially Yoga, Advaita Vedanta and Tantra.

The Three Bodies

Karana Sarira - Causal Body

Karana sarira or the causal body is merely the cause or seed of the subtle body and the gross body. It has no other function than being the seed of the subtle and the gross body. It is *nirvikalpa rupam*, "undifferentiated form". It originates with *avidya*, "ignorance" or "nescience" of the real identity of the atman, instead giving birth to the notion of *jiva*.

Swami Sivananda characterizes the causal body as "The beginningless ignorance that is indescribable". Siddharameshwar Maharaj, the guru of Nisargadatta Maharaj, also describes the causal body as characterized by "emptiness", "ignorance", and "darkness". In the search for the "I am", this is a state where there is nothing to hold on to anymore.

Ramanuja concludes that it is at this stage that consummation of the atman with the Paramatman is reached and the search for the highest Purusa, i.e., of Ishvara, ends.

According to other philosophical schools, the causal body is not the *atman*, because it also has a beginning and an end and is subject to modification. Shankara, not seeking a personal god, goes beyond *Anandamaya Kosha* in search of the transcendent Brahman.

The Indian tradition identifies it with the *Anandamaya kosha*, and the deep sleep state, where *buddhi* becomes dormant and all concepts of time fail, although there are differences between these three descriptions.

The causal body is considered as the most complex of the three bodies. It contains the impressions of experience, which results from past experience.

Suksma Sarira - Subtle Body

Suksma sarira or the subtle body is the body of the mind and the vital energies, which keep the physical body alive. Together with the causal body it is the transmigrating soul or jiva, separating from the gross body upon death.

The subtle body is composed of the five subtle elements, the elements before they have undergone panchikarana, and contains:

- *sravanadipanchakam* - the five organs of perception: eyes, ears, skin, tongue and nose,
- *vagadipanchakam* - the five organs of action: speech, hands, legs, anus and genitals,

- *pranapanchakam* - the five-fold vital breath: Prana (respiration), Apana (evacuation of waste from the body), Vyana (blood circulation), Udana (actions like sneezing, crying, vomiting etc), Samana (digestion),
- manas,
- Buddhi, the Intellect, discriminating wisdom.

Other Indian traditions see the subtle body as an eighth-fold aggregate, placing together the mind-aspects and adding avidhya, kamah and karma:

- *buddhyadicatustayam* (*buddhi, manas, ahamkrti, citta*),
- *avidya* (*adhyasa*, super-imposition),
- *kamah* (desire),
- *karma* (action of the nature of *dharma* and *adharma*).

In samkhya, which does not acknowledge a causal body, it is also known as the *linga-sarira*. It puts one in the mind of the *atman*, it reminds one of the *atman*, the controller. It is the beginning-less limitation of the *atman*, it has no beginning like the *Sthula sarira*.

The "dream state" is a distinct state of the subtle body, where the *buddhi* shines itself owing to memory of deeds done in the waking state. It is the indispensable operative cause of all the activities of the individual self.

Sthula Sarira - Gross Body

Sthula sarira or the gross body is the material physical mortal body that eats, breathes and moves (acts). It is composed of many diverse components, produced by one's *karmas* (actions) in past life out of the elements which have undergone *panchikarana* i.e. combining of the five primordial subtle elements.

It is the instrument of Jiva's experience, which, attached to the body and dominated by *Ahamkara*, uses the body's external and internal organs of sense and action. The Jiva, identifying itself with the body, in its waking state enjoys gross objects. On its body rests man's contact with the external world.

The *Sthula sarira*'s main features are *Sambhava* (birth), *Jara* (old age or ageing) and *Maranam* (death), and the "Waking State". The *Sthula sarira* is the anatman. The gross bodies, the subtle bodies and the causal worlds make one vast universe.

Correlations with Other Models

Three Bodies and Five Sheaths

The Taittiriya Upanishad describes five koshas, which are also often equated with the three bodies. The three bodies are often equated with the five koshas (sheaths), which cover the atman:

1. *Sthula sarira*, the Gross body, also called the *Annamaya Kosha*.

2. *Suksma sarir'*, the Subtle body, composed of:
    1. *Pranamaya Kosha* (Vital breath or Energy),
    2. *Manomaya Kosha* (Mind),
    3. *Vijnanamaya Kosha* (Intellect).
3. *Karana sarira*, the Causal body, the *Anandamaya Kosha* (Bliss).

Four States of Consciousness and Turiya

The Mandukya Upanishad describes four states of consciousness, namely waking consciousness, dream, and deep sleep, and turiya, the base-consciousness. Waking consciousness, dream, and deep sleep are equated with the three bodies, while turiya is a fourth state, which is equated with atman and purusha.

Turiya

Turiya, pure consciousness, is the fourth state. It is the background that underlies and transcends the three common states of consciousness. In this consciousness both absolute and relative, Saguna Brahman and Nirguna Brahman, are transcended. It is the true state of experience of the infinite (*ananta*) and non-different (*advaita/abheda*), free from the dualistic experience which results from the attempts to conceptualise (*vipalka*) reality. It is the state in which ajativada, non-origination, is apprehended.

Four Bodies

Siddharameshwar Maharaj, the guru of Nisargadatta Maharaj, discerns four bodies, by including turiya or the "Great-Causal Body" as a fourth body. Here resides the knowledge of "I am" that cannot be described, the state before Ignorance and Knowledge, or Turiya state.

Integral Theory

The three bodies are a critical component of Ken Wilber's Integral Theory.

Application in Indian Philosophy

Yoga Physiology

The three bodies are an essential part of the Yoga physiology. Yoga aims at controlling the vital energies of the bodies, thereby attaining siddhis (magical powers) and moksha.

Atma Vijnana

According to the Advaita Vedanta tradition, knowledge of the "self" or atman can be gained by self-inquiry, investigating the three bodies, and disidentifying from them. It is a method which is well-known from Ramana Maharshi, but also from Nisargadatta Maharaj and his teacher Siddharameshwar Maharaj.

By subsequently identifying with the three lower bodies, investigating them, and discarding identification with them when it has become clear that they are not the "I", the sense of "I am" beyond knowledge and Ignorance becomes clearly established.

In this investigation the three bodies are recognized as not being anatman.

Theosophy

The later Theosophists speak of seven bodies or levels of existence that include *Sthula sarira* and *Linga sarira.*

Kosha

A Kosha (also Kosa; Sanskrit कोश, IAST: kośa), usually rendered "sheath", is a covering of the Atman, or Self according to Vedantic philosophy. There are five Koshas, and they are often visualised as the layers of an onion.

Origins

The five sheaths (pancha-kosas) are described in the Taittiriya Upanishad. From gross to fine they are:

1. Annamaya kosha, "foodstuff" sheath (Anna).
2. Pranamaya kosha, "energy" sheath (Prana/apana).
3. Manomaya kosha "mind-stuff" sheath (Manas).
4. Vijnanamaya kosha, "wisdom" sheath (*Vijnana*).
5. Anandamaya kosha, "bliss" sheath (*Ananda*).

According to Vedanta the wise person, being aware of the subtle influences of the five elements within each kosha, ever discerns the Self amidst appearances.

The Five Sheaths

Annamaya Kosha

This is the sheath of the physical self, named from the fact that it is nourished by food. Living through this layer man identifies himself with a mass of skin, flesh, fat, bones, and filth, while the man of discrimination knows his own self, the only reality that there is, as distinct from the body.

Pranamaya Kosha

Pranamaya means composed of prana, the vital principle, the force that vitalizes and holds together the body and the mind. It pervades the whole organism, its one physical manifestation is the breath. As long as this vital principle exists in the organisms, life continues. Coupled with the five organs of action it forms the vital sheath. In the Vivekachudamani it is a modification of vayu or air, it enters into and comes out of the body.

Manomaya Kosha

Manomaya means composed of manas or mind. The mind (manas) along with the five sensory organs is said to constitute the manomaya kosa. The *manomaya kosa*, or "mind-sheath" is said more truly to approximate to personhood than *annamaya kosa* and *pranamaya kosha*. It is the cause of diversity, of *I* and *mine*. Sankara likens it to clouds that are brought in by the wind and again driven away by the same agency. Similarly, man's bondage is caused by the mind, and liberation, too, is caused by that alone.

Vijnanamaya Kosha

Vijnanamaya means composed of vijnana, or intellect, the faculty which discriminates, determines or wills. Chattampi Swamikal defines vijnanamaya as the combination of intellect and the five sense organs. It is the sheath composed of more intellection, associated with the organs of perception. Sankara holds that the buddhi, with its modifications and the organs of knowledge, form the cause of man's transmigration. This knowledge sheath, which seems to be followed by a reflection of the power of the cit, is a modification of prakrti. It is endowed with the function of knowledge and identifies itself with the body, organs etc.

This knowledge sheath cannot be the supreme self for the following reasons;

- It is subject to change.
- It is insentient.
- It is a limited thing.
- It is not constantly present.

Anandamaya Kosha

Anandamaya means composed of ananda, or bliss. In the Upanishads the sheath is known also as the *causal body*. In deep sleep, when the mind and senses cease functioning, it still stands between the finite world and the self. Anandamaya, or that which is composed of Supreme bliss, is regarded as the innermost of all. The bliss sheath normally has its fullest play during deep sleep: while in the dreaming and wakeful states, it has only a partial manifestation. The blissful sheath (anandamaya kosha) is a reflection of the Atman which is truth, beauty, bliss absolute.

The following entry is for the utility of Hindu aspirants who are familiar with Panchakosha:

Just as each of the five elements (earth, water, fire, air, and ether) appear in corresponding subtlety among each of the five senses so too the intellect cognizes ever subtler causes and effects at play through each of the five sheaths.

For example, the annamayakosha, the coarsest sheath, is based in the earth element, which is guarded by Ganesha, while the very subtlest sheath Anandamaya is based in the quanta/ether element, and is guarded by a black disc of utter darkness over the sun, which can be removed only by Ganesha.

Awareness of that reflection of atman/self within the most subtle sheath, Anandamayakosha, however, is but the foundation for discerning that which the elements, energies, senses, and kosha serve. To that end, one re-examines the components of the five koshas in daily devotional meditation after recitation of twenty-one OM, viz, one OM per each of the five elements, the five pranas, the five indriyas, and the five kosha, equaling twenty OM, then a twenty-first OM is offered for the ineffable, such that a spiritual discernment of ever-increasing subtlety arises in the purified intellect, alaya nirvijnana, the womb of the tathagata, wherein silence ensues and clarity blossoms.

Chakra

In Hinduism, Jainism and Buddhism, a chakra (Sanskrit: *Cakra*, Pali : *Cakka*, Tamil: *chakra*) is thought to be an energy point or node in the subtle body. Chakras are believed to be part of the subtle body, not the physical body, and as such, are the meeting points of the subtle (non-physical) energy channels called nadi. Nadi are believed to be channels in the subtle body through which the life force (prana) (non-physical) or vital energy (non-physical) moves. Various scriptural texts and teachings present a different number of chakras. It's believed that there are many chakras in the subtle human body, according to the tantric texts, but there are seven chakras that are considered to be the most important ones.

Etymology

The word Chakra derives from the Sanskrit word meaning "wheel," as well as "circle" and "cycle". It's described by many as a spinning wheel of light. Of the many chakras within the human body, seven have been identified as major.

M. N. Roy's review of tantric history says that the word *chakra* is used to mean several different things in the Sanskrit sources:

1. "Circle," used in a variety of senses, symbolising endless rotation of shakti.
2. A circle of people. In rituals, there are different *cakrasādhanā*s in which adherents assemble and perform rites. According to the *Niruttaratantra*, chakras in the sense of assemblies are of 5 types.
3. The term chakra is also used to denote yantras (mystic diagram)s, variously known as *trikoṇa-cakra*, *aṣṭakoṇa-cakra*, etc.
4. Different nerve plexuses within the body.

In Buddhism, the Sanskrit term *cakra* (Pali *cakka*) is used in a different sense of "circle," referring to the conception of rebirth consisting of six states in which beings may be reborn.

History

Breath channels (nāḍi) of yogic practices are mentioned in the classical Upanishads, but hierarchies of chakras are introduced in the eighth-century Buddhist Hevajra Tantra and *Caryāgiti*.

Characteristics

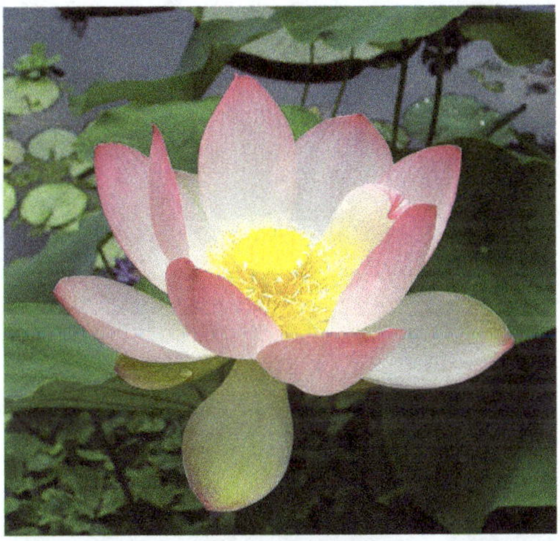

Chakras (as well as Yantras and Mandalas) are visualised as lotus with different number of petals representing each chakra.

The texts and teachings present different numbers of chakras. Also, different physical structures are considered chakras. David Gordon White thus emphasises:

"In fact, there is no "standard" system of the *chakras*. Every school, sometimes every teacher within each school, has had his own *chakra* system."

The following features are common:

- They form part of the body, along with the breath channels (nadi), and the winds (vayu).
- They are located along the central channel (sushumna/avadhūtī).
- Two side channels cross the centre channel at the location of the chakras.
- They possess a number of 'petals' or 'spokes'.
- They are generally associated with a mantra seed-syllable, and often with a variety of colours and deities.
- There are believed to be 7 major chakras.

Use in Eastern Traditions

Hindu Tantra

David Gordon White traces the modern popularity of the "Hindu" seven chakra system to Arthur Avalon's *The Serpent Power*, which was Avalon's translation of a late work, the *Satcakranirupana*.

In actuality, there are several models and systems present in Hindu tantric literature, as White documents. Kundalini is a feature of Hindu chakra systems.

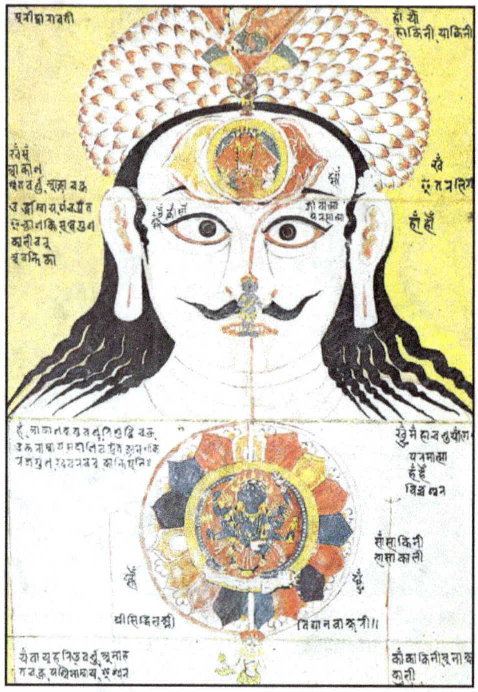

Thousand Petalled lotus Crown, Two Petalled Brow Chakra, Sixteen Petalled Throat Chakra (Nepal, 17th Century).

Vajrayana

Chakras play an important role in the main surviving branch of Indian Vajrayana, Tibetan Buddhism. They play a pivotal role in completion stage practices, where an attempt is made to bring the subtle winds of the body into the central channel, to realise the clear light of bliss and emptiness, and to attain Buddhahood.

The Vajrayana system states that the central channel (avadhūtī) begins at the point of the third eye like of lord Shiva, curves up to the crown of the head, and then goes straight down to the lower body. There are two side channels, the rasanā and lalanā, which start at their respective nostrils and then travel down to the lower body. The apāna vāyu governs the lower terminations of the three channels. The lower end of the central channel ends in the rectum. The lower end of the lalanā ends in the urinary tract. The lower end of the rasanā channel emits semen.

The side channels run parallel to the centre channel, except at locations such as the navel, heart, throat and crown (i.e. chakras) where the two side channels twist around the central channel. At the navel, throat and crown, there is a twofold knot caused by each side channel twisting once around the central channel. At the heart wheel there is a sixfold knot, where each side channel twists around three times. An important part of completion stage practice involves loosening and undoing these knots.

Within the chakras exist the 'subtle drops'. The white drop exists in the crown, the red drop exists in the navel, and at the heart exists the indestructible red and white drop, which leaves the body at the time of death. In addition, each chakra has a number of 'spokes' or 'petals', which branch off into thousands of subtle channels running to every part of the body, and each contains a Sanskrit syllable.

By focusing on a specific chakra (while often holding the breath) the subtle winds enter the central channel. The chakra at which they enter is important in order to realise specific practices. For example, focusing on the subnavel area is important for the practice of tummo, or inner fire. Meditating on the heart chakra is important for realising clear light. Meditating on the throat chakra is important for lucid dreaming and the practices of dream yoga. And meditating on the crown chakra is important for consciousness projection, either to another world, or into another body.

A result of energetic imbalance among the chakras is an almost continuous feeling of dissatisfaction. When the heart chakra is agitated, people lose touch with feelings and sensations, and that breeds the sense of dissatisfaction. That leads to looking outside for fulfilment. When people live in their heads, feelings are secondary; they are interpretations of mental images that are fed back to the individual. When awareness is focused on memories of past experiences and mental verbalisations, the energy flow to the head chakra increases and the energy flow to the heart chakra lessens. Without nurturing feelings of the heart a subtle form of anxiety arises which results in the self reaching out for experience. When the throat chakra settles and energy is distributed evenly between the head and the heart chakras, one is able to truly contact one's senses and touch real feelings.

Bön

Chakras, according to the Bon tradition, influence the quality of experience, because movement of vayu cannot be separated from experience. Each of the six major chakras is linked to experiential qualities of one of the six realms of existence.

A modern teacher, Tenzin Wangyal Rinpoche, uses a computer analogy: main chakras are like hard drives. Each hard drive has many files. One of the files is always open in each of the chakras, no matter how "closed" that particular chakra may be. What is displayed by the file shapes experience.

The tsa lung practices such as those embodied in Trul khor lineages open channels so *lung* (the Tibetan term for vayu) may move without obstruction. Yoga opens chakras and evokes positive qualities associated with a particular chakra. In the hard drive analogy, the screen is cleared and a file is called up that contains positive, supportive qualities. A bīja (seed syllable) is used both as a password that evokes the positive quality and the armour that sustains the quality.

Tantric practice is said to eventually transform all experience into bliss. The practice aims to liberate from negative conditioning and leads to control over perception and cognition.

Qigong

Qigong (氣功) also relies on a similar model of the human body as an esoteric energy system, except that it involves the circulation of qì (氣, also *ki*) or life-energy. The qì, equivalent to the Hindu prana, flows through the energy channels called meridians, equivalent to the nadi, but two other energies are also important: *jīng*, or primordial essence, and *shén*, or spirit energy.

In the principle circuit of qì, called the microcosmic orbit, energy rises up a main meridian along the spine, but also comes back down the front torso. Throughout its cycle it enters various dantian (elixir fields) which act as furnaces, where the types of energy in the body (jing, qi and shen) are progressively refined. These dantian play a very similar role to that of chakras. The number of dantian varies depending on the system; the navel dantian is the most well-known, but there is usually a dantian located at the heart and between the eyebrows. The lower dantian at or below the navel transforms essence, or jīng, into qì. The middle dantian in the middle of the chest transforms qì into shén, or spirit, and the higher dantian at the level of the forehead (or at the top of the head), transforms shen into wuji, infinite space of void.

Indonesian and Malaysian Metaphysics

Traditional spirituality in the Malay Archipelago borrows heavily from Hindu-Buddhist concepts. In Malay and Indonesian metaphysical theory, the chakras' energy rotates outwards along diagonal lines. Defensive energy emits outwards from the centre line, while offensive energy moves inwards from the sides of the body. This can be applied to energy-healing, meditation, or martial arts. Silat practitioners learn to harmonise their movements with the chakras, thereby increasing the power and effectiveness of attacks and movements.

Western Interpretations

Western Adaptation of Hindu Yogic Chakras

In Western culture, a concept similar to that of prana can be traced back as far as the 18th century's Franz Anton Mesmer, who used "animal magnetism" to treat disease.

However, it was only in 1918 that the shakta theory of seven main chakras, that has become most popular in the West, was introduced, largely through the translation of two Indian texts: the *Sat-Cakra-Nirupana* and the *Padaka-Pancaka*, by Sir John Woodroffe, alias Arthur Avalon, in a book titled *The Serpent Power*.

This book is extremely detailed and complex, and later the ideas were developed into the predominant Western view of the chakras by C. W. Leadbeater in his book *The Chakras*. Many of the views which directed Leadbeater's understanding of the chakras were influenced by previous theosophist authors, in particular Johann Georg Gichtel, a disciple of Jakob Böhme, and his book *Theosophia Practica (1696)*, in which Gichtel directly refers to inner *force centres*, a concept reminiscent of the chakras.

Hesychasm

A completely separate contemplative movement within the Eastern Orthodox Church is Hesychasm, a form of Christian meditation. Comparisons have been made between the Hesychastic centres of prayer and the position of the chakras. Particular emphasis is placed upon the heart area. However, there is no talk about these centres as having any sort of metaphysical existence. Far more than in any of the cases discussed above, the centres are simply places to focus the concentration during prayer.

New Age

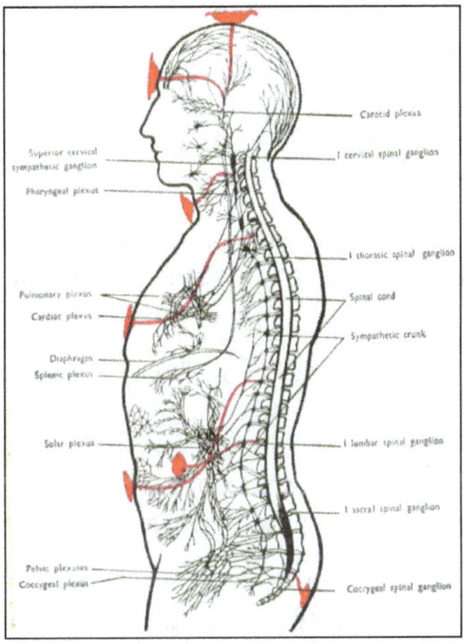

Chakra positions in relation to nervous plexi.

In *Anatomy of the Spirit* (1996), Caroline Myss describes the function of chakras as follows: "Every thought and experience you've ever had in your life gets filtered through these chakra databases. Each event is recorded into your cells...". The chakras are described as being aligned in an ascending column from the base of the spine to the top of the head. New Age practices often associate each chakra with a certain colour. In various traditions, chakras are associated with multiple physiological functions, an aspect of consciousness, a classical element, and other distinguishing characteristics. They are visualised as lotuses or flowers with a different number of petals in every chakra.

The chakras are thought to vitalise the physical body and to be associated with interactions of a physical, emotional and mental nature. They are considered loci of life energy or prana (which New Age belief equates with *shakti*, *qi* in Chinese, *ki* in Japanese, *koach-ha-guf* in Hebrew, *bios* in Greek, and *aether* in both Greek and English), which is thought to flow among them along pathways called nadi. The function of the chakras is to spin and draw in this energy to keep the spiritual, mental, emotional and physical health of the body in balance.

In his book on Japa Yoga (Himalaya Press, 1978), Swami Sivananda states that a yogi that practices Japa only with the Om and is successful at Mahasamyama (oneness with the object —in this case, a word being meditated on—) becomes a direct disciple of the Om, the most holy of all words and syllables (the same as the word of creation as recognised by the Torah, although this is not professed or quite possibly not even recognised by those of secular authority in either Judaism or Christianity). Thus, the yogi who achieves this feat needs no guru or Sat-guru to achieve any spiritual goal (an archetype or an Ascended Master —a Krishna, a Rama, a Jesus, a Nanak, a Buddha...—). Swami Sivananda mentions that this yogi has a path that is, in all recognisable ways and manners, reverse of that of other yogis or spiritual aspirants and their paths, in that this spiritual aspirant then works through the chakras, mastering them from the crown down. Satprem explains, in page 67 of his book *Sri Aurobindo, or the Adventure of Consciousness* (ISBN 81-85137-60-9), that, in

Sri Aurobindo and the Mother's Integral Yoga, the practitioner experiences a "descent" where the Grace and Light works through and enlightens the chakras from the crown chakra downwards.

Another interpretation of the seven chakras is presented by writer and artist Zachary Selig. In his book *Kundalini Awakening, a Gentle Guide to Chakra Activation and Spiritual Growth,* he presents a unique codex titled "Relaxatia", a solar Kundalini paradigm that is a codex of the human chakra system and the solar light spectrum, designed to activate Kundalini through his colour-coded chakra paintings.

Some system models describe one or more transpersonal chakras above the crown chakra, as well as an Earth star chakra below the feet. There are also held to be many minor chakras (for example, between the major chakras).

Rudolf Steiner considered the chakra system to be dynamic and evolving. He suggested that this system has become different for modern people than it was in ancient times and that it will, in turn, be radically different in future times. Steiner described a sequence of development that begins with the upper chakras and moves down, rather than moving in the opposite direction. He gave suggestions on how to develop the chakras through disciplining thoughts, feelings, and will.

According to Florin Lowndes, a "spiritual student" can further develop and deepen or elevate thinking consciousness when taking the step from the "ancient path" of schooling to the "new path" represented by Steiner's *The Philosophy of Freedom.*

Endocrine System

Chakras and their importance are posited to reside in the psyche. However, there are those who believe that chakras have a physical manifestation as well. Gary Osborn, for instance, has described the chakras as metaphysical counterparts to the endocrine glands, while Anodea Judith noted a marked similarity between the positions of the two and the roles described for each. Stephen Sturgess also links the lower six chakras to specific nerve plexuses along the spinal cord as well as glands. C.W. Leadbeater associated the Ajna chakra with the pineal gland, which is a part of the endocrine system. These associations remain speculative, however, and have yet to be empirically validated.

Spectrum of Light

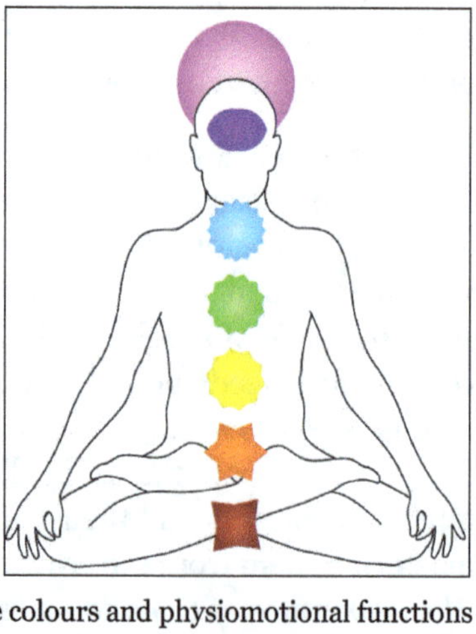

Recent Western traditions associate colours and physiomotional functions for each of the seven main chakras.

A development in Western practices dating back to the 1940s is to associate each one of the seven chakras to a given colour and a corresponding crystal. For example, the chakra in the forehead is associated with the colour purple, so to try and cure a headache a person might apply a purple stone to the forehead.

Mercier introduces the relation of colour energy to the science of the light spectrum:

As humans, we exist within the 49th Octave of Vibration of the electromagnetic light spectrum. Below this range are barely visible radiant heat, then invisible infrared, television and radiowaves, sound and brain waves; above it is barely visible ultraviolet, then the invisible frequencies of chemicals and perfumes, followed by x-rays, gamma rays, radium rays and unknown cosmic rays.

Understanding existence and physical form as an interpretation of light energy through the physical eyes will open up greater potential to explore the energetic boundaries of colour, form and light that are perceived as immediate reality. Indian Yogic teachings assign to the seven major chakras specific qualities, such as colour of influence (from the seven rays of spectrum light), elements (such as earth, air, water & ether), body sense (such as touch, taste, and smell), and relation to an endocrine gland.

Description of Each Chakra

There are believed to be seven major chakras, which are arranged vertically along the axial channel (sushumna nadi). David Gordon White traces the modern popularity of the seven chakra system to Arthur Avalon's *The Serpent Power,* which was Avalon's translation of a late work, the *Sat-Cakra-Nirupana*. Below is a description of the seven chakras, with various associations. Each of these chakras also has its elemental deity (Vasu), demigod of its material element.

From the top down, they are thought to be:

Sahasrara

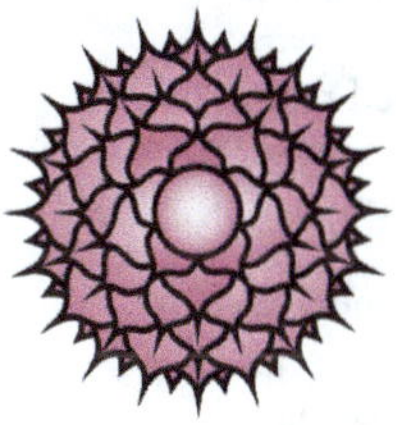

Sahasrara (Sanskrit: सहस्रार, IAST: Sahasrāra, English: "thousand-petaled") or crown chakra is generally considered to be the state of pure consciousness, within which there is neither object nor subject. When the Kundalini energy rises to this point, it unites with the male Shiva energy, and a state of liberating samadhi is attained. Symbolized by a lotus with one thousand multi-coloured petals, it is located either at the crown of the head, or above the crown of the head. Sahasrara is represented by the colour white and it involves such issues as inner wisdom and the death of the body.

Its role may be envisioned somewhat similarly to that of the pituitary gland, which secretes hormones to communicate to the rest of the endocrine system and also connects to the central nervous system via the hypothalamus. According to Gary Osborn, the thalamus is thought to have a key role in the physical basis of consciousness and is the 'Bridal Chamber' mentioned in the Gnostic scriptures. Sahasrara's inner aspect deals with the release of karma, physical action with meditation, mental action with universal consciousness and unity, and emotional action with "beingness."

In Tibetan Buddhism, the point at the crown of the head is represented by a white circle, with 33 downward pointing petals. It is of primary importance in the performance of phowa, or consciousness projection after death, in order to obtain rebirth in a Pure Land. Within this state is contained the White drop, or Bodhicitta, which is the essence of masculine energy.

Corresponding deity for material element of this state is Dhruva.
The tone is 172.06 Hz = F.

Ajna

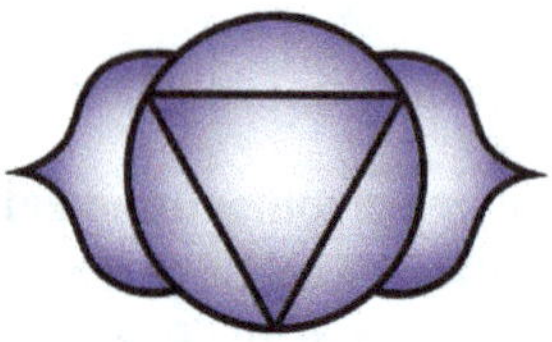

Ajna (Sanskrit: आज्ञा, IAST: Ājñā, English: "command") or third-eye chakra is symbolised by a lotus with two petals, and corresponds to the colours violet, indigo or deep blue, though it is traditionally described as white. It is at this point that the two side nadi Ida (yoga) and Pingala are said to terminate and merge with the central channel Sushumna, signifying the end of duality, the characteristic of being dual (e.g. *light* and *dark*, or *male* and *female*). The seed syllable for this chakra is the syllable OM, and the presiding deity is Ardhanarishvara, who is a half male, half female Shiva/Shakti. The Shakti goddess of Ajna is called Hakini.

Ajna (along with Bindu), is known as the third eye chakra and is linked to the pineal gland which may inform a model of its envisioning. The pineal gland is a light sensitive gland that produces the hormone melatonin which regulates sleep and waking up, and is also postulated to be the production site of the psychedelic dimethyltryptamine, the only known hallucinogen endogenous to the human body. Ajna's key issues involve balancing the higher and lower selves and trusting inner guidance. Ajna's inner aspect relates to the access of intuition. Mentally, Ajna deals with visual consciousness. Emotionally, Ajna deals with clarity on an intuitive level.

The tone is 221.23 Hz = A.

Vishuddha

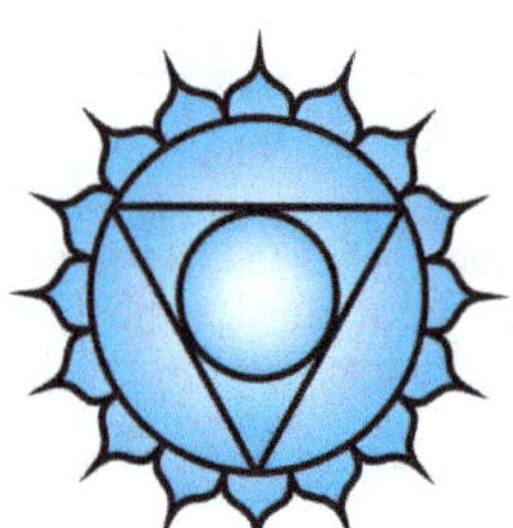

Vishuddha (Sanskrit: विशुद्ध, IAST: Viśuddha, English: "especially pure"), or Vishuddhi, or throat chakra is depicted as a silver crescent within a white circle, with 16 light or pale blue, or turquoise petals. The seed mantra is Ham, and the residing deity is Panchavaktra shiva, with 5 heads and 4 arms, and the Shakti is Shakini.

Vishuddha may be understood as relating to communication and growth through expression. This chakra is paralleled to the thyroid, a gland that is also in the throat and which produces thyroid hormone, responsible for growth and maturation. Physically, Vishuddha governs communication, emotionally it governs independence, mentally it governs fluent thought, and spiritually, it governs a sense of security.

In Tibetan buddhism, this chakra is red, with 16 upward pointing petals. It plays an important role in Dream Yoga, the art of lucid dreaming.

Corresponding deity for material element of this chakra is Dyaus.

The tone is 141.27 Hz = C#.

Anahata

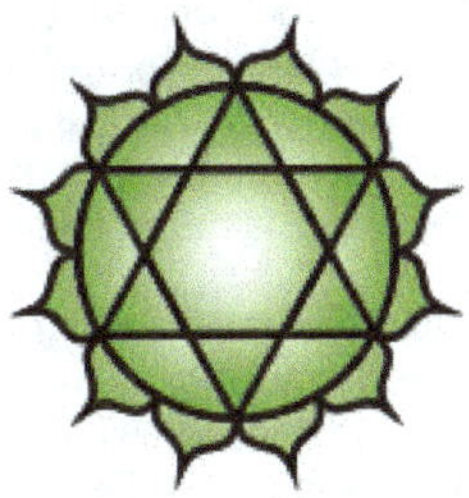

Anahata (Sanskrit: अनाहत, IAST: Anāhata, English: "unstruck") or heart chakra is symbolised by a circular flower with twelve green petals called the heartmind. Within it is a yantra of two intersecting triangles, forming a hexagram, symbolising a union of the male and female. The seed mantra is Yam, the presiding deity is Ishana Rudra Shiva, and the Shakti is Kakini.

Anahata is related to the thymus, located in the chest. The thymus is an element of the immune system as well as being part of the endocrine system. It is the site of maturation of the T cells responsible for fending off disease and may be adversely affected by stress. Anahata is related to the colours green or pink. Key issues involving Anahata involve complex emotions, compassion, tenderness, unconditional love, equilibrium, rejection and well-being. Physically Anahata governs circulation, emotionally it governs unconditional love for the self and others, mentally it governs passion, and spiritually it governs devotion.

The tone is 136.10 Hz = C#.

Manipura

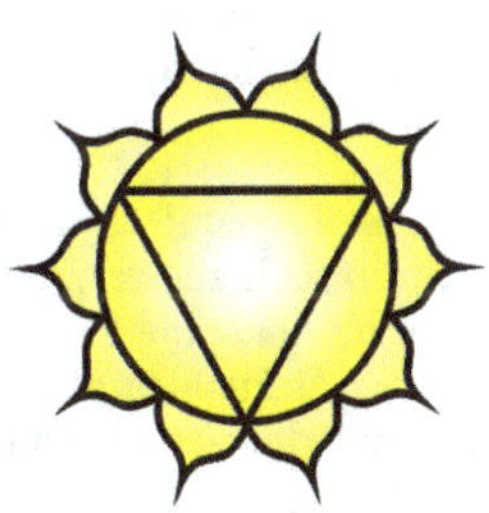

Manipura (Sanskrit: मणिपूर, IAST: Maṇipūra, English: "jewel city") or solar plexus/navel chakra is symbolised by a downward pointing triangle with ten petals, along with the colour yellow. The seed syllable is Ram, and the presiding deity is Braddha Rudra, with Lakini as the Shakti.

Manipura is related to the metabolic and digestive systems. Manipura is believed to correspond to Islets of Langerhans, which are groups of cells in the pancreas, as well as the outer adrenal glands and the adrenal cortex. These play a valuable role in digestion, the conversion of food matter into energy for the body. The colour that corresponds to Manipura is yellow. Key issues governed by Manipura are issues of personal power, fear, anxiety, opinion-formation, introversion, and transition from simple or base emotions to complex. Physically, Manipura governs digestion, mentally it governs personal power, emotionally it governs expansiveness, and spiritually, all matters of growth.

Corresponding deity for material element of this chakra is Agni.

The tone is 126.22 Hz = B.

Svadhishthana

Svadhishthana (Sanskrit: स्वाधिष्ठान, IAST: Svādhiṣṭhāna, English: "one's own base") or sacral chakra is symbolised by a white lotus within which is a crescent moon, with six vermilion, or orange petals. The seed mantra is Vam, and the presiding deity is Brahma, with the Shakti being Rakini (or Chakini). The animal associated is the crocodile of Varuna.

This chakra is located in the sacrum and is considered to correspond to the testes or the ovaries that produce the various sex hormones involved in the reproductive cycle. Svadhishthana is also considered to be related to, more generally, the genitourinary system and the adrenals. The key issues involving Svadhishthana are relationships, violence, addictions, basic emotional needs, and pleasure. Physically, Svadhishthana governs reproduction, mentally it governs creativity, emotionally it governs joy, and spiritually it governs enthusiasm.

The tone is 210.42 Hz = G#.

Muladhara

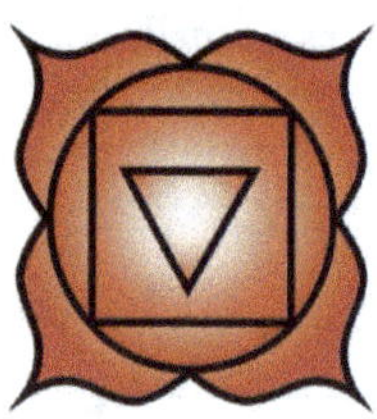

Muladhara (Sanskrit: मूलाधार, IAST: Mūlādhāra, English: "root support") or root chakra is symbolised by a lotus with four petals and the colour red. This centre is located at the base of the spine in the coccygeal region. It is said to relate to the gonads and the adrenal medulla, responsible for the fight-or-flight response when survival is under threat. The seed syllable is LAM.

Muladhara is related to instinct, security, survival and also to basic human potentiality. Physically, Muladhara governs sexuality, mentally it governs stability, emotionally it governs sensuality, and spiritually it governs a sense of security. Muladhara also has a relation to the sense of smell.

This chakra is where the three main nadi separate and begin their upward movement. Dormant Kundalini rests here, wrapped three and a half times around the black Svayambhu linga, the lowest of three obstructions to her full rising (also known as knots or granthis). It is the seat of the red bindu, the female drop (which in Tibetan vajrayana is located at the navel chakra).

The seed syllable is Lam (pronounced *lum*), the deity is Ganesh, and the Shakti is Dakini. The associated animal is the elephant.

The tone is 194.18 Hz = G .

Other Chakras

Hridhiya chakra (also known as *hrid chakra*) is measured from centre of Anahata chakra, two fingers to the left and continue with two finger down, whereby the heart beat can be felt. Talu chakra is located at behind of Reticular Formation at Fourth Ventrical before beginning of spinal cord. There are said to be 21 minor chakras which are reflected points of the major chakras. These 21 are further grouped into ten bilateral minor chakras that correspond to the foot, hand, knee, elbow, groin, clavicle, navel, shoulder and ear. The spleen may also be listed by some authorities as a location for a minor chakra.

Secret Chakras

There are said to be three chakras that are beyond the physical and spiritual. They are called Golata, Lalata, and Lalana and "located on the uvula at the back of the throat, above the Ajna chakra, and within the soft upper palate". According to Robert Svoboda they defy description in the sense of the above seven and can only be experienced once Kundalini has fully awakened.

Minor Chakras Below Muladhara

There are said to be a series of seven chakras below Muladhara going down the leg, corresponding the base animal instincts, and to the Hindu underworld patala. From the top down they are:

Atala – Located in the hips, it governs fear and lust.

Vitala – Located in the thighs, it governs anger and resentment.

Sutala – Located in the knees, it governs jealousy.

Talatala – Translated as "under the bottom level", it is located in the calves and represents a state of prolonged confusion and instinctive wilfulness.

Rasatala – Located in the ankles, it is the centre of selfishness and pure animal nature.

Mahatala – Located in the feet, this is the dark realm 'without conscience', and inner blindness.

Patala – Located in the soles of the feet, this is the realm of malice, murder, torture and hatred, and in Hindu mythology it borders on the realm of Naraka, or hell.

Nadi

Nadi (pronounced [ˈnandi]) is the third-largest conurbation in Fiji. It is located on the western side of the main island of Viti Levu, and had a population of 42,284 at the most recent census, in 2007. A 2012 estimate showed that the population had grown to over 50,000. Nadi is multiracial with many of its inhabitants Indian or Fijian, along with a large transient population of foreign tourists. Along with sugar cane production, tourism is a mainstay of the local economy.

With its large Indo-Fijian population, Nadi is a centre for Hinduism and Islam in Fiji. The downtown area is defined by the Nadi River and Viseisei village on the west side, and the Sri Siva Subramaniya temple on the east. It is the largest Hindu temple in the Southern hemisphere, and is a site for pilgrims. Nadi International Airport located 9 kilometres from the town, is the largest airport in Fiji. Thus, Nadi is the principal port of entry for air travellers to Fiji, even though it is on the opposite (western) side of the island of Viti Levu from the nation's capital and largest city, Suva.

History

Nadi Township was established in 1947. Around that time the colonial government of Fiji established offices on the higher grounds of Nadi. A few businesses were then established around the government offices to service them, and other business organisations from other parts of Fiji followed suit. Some concerned citizens of Nadi attempted to move the town centre to Martintar because the existing centre was prone to flooding, but this did not eventuate because the move Nadi Township had already developed strong roots in its existing location.

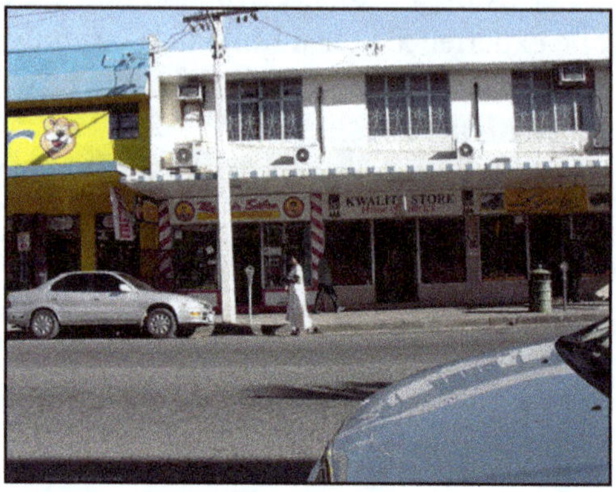

Part of Main Street in Nadi.

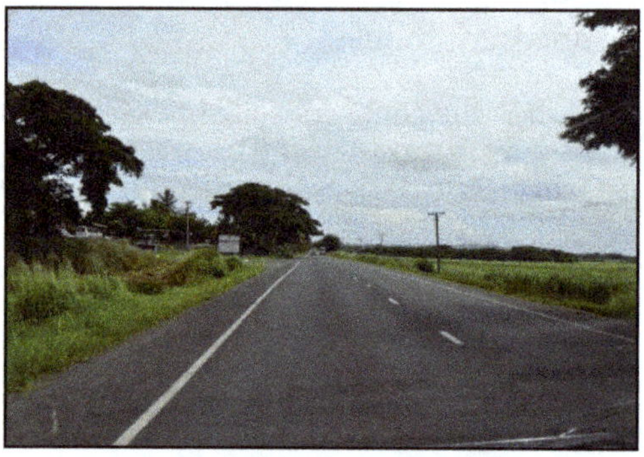

Tarsealed road outside Nadi.

Elective local government was introduced in 1967. Dr A. H. Sahu Khan was the first elected Chairman of the Nadi Township Board. With the introduction of the Local Government Act in 1972, the status of the Board was changed to a Town Council. H. M. Lodhia became the first Mayor of Nadi in 1972 and remained in office until December 1973. The most recent Mayor of Nadi was Councillor S. Sami. At present, elected municipal government in Nadi (and also throughout Fiji) is suspended, and government-appointed Administrators are carrying out the functions normally fulfilled by the City Council.

Government and Infrastructure

The Civil Aviation Authority of Fiji (CAAFI) head office is at Nadi Airport in Nadi.

Economy

Fiji Airways, formerly Air Pacific has its head office at the Air Pacific Maintenance & Administration Centre at Nadi International Airport in Nadi. Fiji Airlines Limited, operating as Pacific Sun, is headquartered in the Pacific Sun building in the Civil Aviation Authority of Fiji (CAAFI) compound at Nadi International Airport.

Climate

Climate data for Nadi, Fiji (1961–1990)													
Month	**Jan**	**Feb**	**Mar**	**Apr**	**May**	**Jun**	**Jul**	**Aug**	**Sep**	**Oct**	**Nov**	**Dec**	**Year**
Record high °C (°F)	36.7 (98.1)	35.4 (95.7)	35.0 (95)	34.3 (93.7)	33.9 (93)	33.5 (92.3)	32.9 (91.2)	34.3 (93.7)	34.0 (93.2)	34.6 (94.3)	36.3 (97.3)	35.9 (96.6)	36.7 (98.1)
Average high °C (°F)	31.6 (88.9)	31.5 (88.7)	31.1 (88)	30.7 (87.3)	29.7 (85.5)	29.2 (84.6)	28.5 (83.3)	28.7 (83.7)	29.4 (84.9)	30.2 (86.4)	30.9 (87.6)	31.4 (88.5)	30.2 (86.4)
Daily mean °C (°F)	27.1 (80.8)	27.2 (81)	26.9 (80.4)	26.2 (79.2)	24.9 (76.8)	24.2 (75.6)	23.4 (74.1)	23.6 (74.5)	24.4 (75.9)	25.3 (77.5)	26.2 (79.2)	26.7 (80.1)	25.5 (77.9)
Average low °C (°F)	22.7 (72.9)	22.9 (73.2)	22.6 (72.7)	21.7 (71.1)	20.1 (68.2)	19.3 (66.7)	18.3 (64.9)	18.4 (65.1)	19.3 (66.7)	20.4 (68.7)	21.5 (70.7)	22.1 (71.8)	20.8 (69.4)
Record low °C (°F)	19.0 (66.2)	18.3 (64.9)	17.7 (63.9)	16.2 (61.2)	14.0 (57.2)	13.6 (56.5)	11.7 (53.1)	11.3 (52.3)	13.3 (55.9)	14.4 (57.9)	15.1 (59.2)	17.2 (63)	11.3 (52.3)
Average rainfall mm (inches)	300 (11.81)	303 (11.93)	324 (12.76)	173 (6.81)	80 (3.15)	62 (2.44)	47 (1.85)	59 (2.32)	77 (3.03)	103 (4.06)	139 (5.47)	159 (6.26)	1,826 (71.89)
Mean monthly sunshine hours	213.5	182.4	190.1	197.8	212.0	206.0	218.1	231.0	214.6	226.6	221.5	225.4	2,539

References

- Gardiner, Philip; Osborn, Gary (2006). The Shining Ones: the world's most powerful secret society revealed (Rev. and updated ed.). London: Watkins. pp. 44–45. ISBN 1-84293-150-4
- Gregory P., Fields (2001). Religious Therapeutics: Body and Health in Yoga, Āyurveda and Tantra. State University of New York Press. p. 27. Retrieved 04, June 2020
- Mercier, Patricia (2007). The Chakra Bible: the definitive guide to working with chakras. London: Godsfield Press/Octopus Publishing. p. 12. ISBN 978-1-84181-320-2
- Ed Hudson (2008-05-01). The Popular Encyclopedia of Apologetics. Harvest House Publishers. p. 471. ISBN 9780736936354
- Tulku, Tarthang (2007). Tibetan relaxation : the illustrated guide to Kum Nye massage and movement-- a yoga from the Tibetan tradition (Rev. ed.). London: Duncan Baird. pp. 31, 33. ISBN 978-1-84483-404-4
- Franco Marcello Antonetti (2012-02-27). The Enigma of God:A Revelation to Man. Balboa Press. p. 32. ISBN 9781452547404
- Wheels of Life: A User's Guide to the Chakra System - Anodea Judith - Google Books. Books.google.com. Retrieved 05,August 2020
- Arvind Sharma (2006-09-09). A Primal Perspective on the philosophy of Religion. Springer. p. 193. ISBN 9781402050145
- Roeser, Robert W. (2005). An introduction to Hindu India's contemplative psychological perspective on motivation, self, and development (PDF) (pdf ed.). p. 15. Retrieved 25, June 2020

- Dahlby, Tenzin Wangyal Rinpoche ; edited by Mark (2002). Healing with Form, Energy, and Light: the five elements in Tibetan Shamanism, Tantra, and Dzogchen. Ithaca, NY: Snow Lion Pub. p. 84. ISBN 1-55939-176-6
- Lowndes, Florin (2000). Enlivening the Chakra of the Heart: The Fundamental Spiritual Exercises of Rudolf Steiner (2nd ed.). London: Sophia Books. ISBN 1-85584-053-7
- Dahlby, Tenzin Wangyal Rinpoche ; edited by Mark (2002). Healing with Form, Energy, and Light: the five elements in Tibetan Shamanism, Tantra, and Dzogchen. Ithaca, NY: Snow Lion Pub. pp. 84–85. ISBN 1-55939-176-6
- Rinpoche, Tenzin Wangyal (2002). Healing with Form, Energy, and Light: the five elements in Tibetan Shamanism, Tantra, and Dzogchen. Ithaca, NY: Snow Lion Pub. pp. 84–85. ISBN 1-55939-176-6

4

Techniques of Yoga

There are various practices and techniques which are an integral part of yoga such as anuyoga, mahayoga, sahaja yoga, asana, mudra, kriyi, yamas, niyama and pratyahara. The aim of this chapter is to explore these practices and techniques of yoga. These topics are crucial for a complete understanding of the subject.

Anuyoga

Anuyoga (Skt. **अनुयोग** 'further yoga') is the designation of the second of the three Inner Tantras according to the ninefold division of practice used by the Nyingma school of Tibetan Buddhism. As with the other yanas, Anuyoga represents both a scriptural division as well as a specific emphasis of both view and practice.

Position in the Nine-yana Schema

Anuyoga is said to emphasise the completion stage of Tantra, where the preceding division, Mahayoga emphasises the generation stage. Dalton (2003: unpaginated) in introducing the literature of the Anuyoga-yana affirms the affiliation of the Anuyoga-yana with the 'completion stage' or the 'perfection stage':

Modern-day doxographical presentations of the Nyingma school are usually based on the system of the nine vehicles (*theg pa dgu*). Emphasis is placed on the highest three vehicles in this scheme, namely Mahāyoga, Anuyoga, and Atiyoga. Generally speaking, these three "inner" yogas correspond to three stages in tantric practice, namely the generation stage, during which the details of the visualizations are stabilised, the perfection stage, in which those visualizations are then employed towards familiarizing oneself with the state of enlightenment, and finally the Great Perfection, the spontaneous accomplishment of buddhahood. Being the second of the three inner yogas, Anuyoga is thus associated with the practices of the perfection stage.

Ray (2002: p. 124-125) mentions visualization, subtle body, chakra, prana, nadis, bindu and pure land:

Anuyoga-yana is associated with the feminine principle and is for those whose principal obstacle is passion. In anuyoga the emphasis shifts away from external visualization toward the completion stage, in which one meditates on the inner or subtle body with its primary energy centres (*chakras*), and its *prana* (winds or subtle energies), *nadis* (the inner pathways along which one's energy travels), and *bindu* (the consciousness). In anuyoga, all appearances are seen as the three great mandalas, and reality is understood as the deities and their pure lands.

Germano (2002: unpaginated) frames the importance of Nub Sangye Yeshe as the instigator of

Anuyoga within Tibet and states that it was: "the late ninth century Nub Sangye Yeshe (gnubs sangs rgyas ye shes), who inaugurated the Anuyoga tradition in Tibet...".

Dudjom (1904-1987), *et al.* (1991: p. 460 History) relate an important source that impacts on the story of King Ja (particularly the narrative of the Buddhadharma relics falling from the sky upon the royal palace) a happenstance which is implied to be concurrent with the emergence of the texts of Anuyoga in Sri Lanka with the provision of a quote of what Dudjom *et al.* identify as a "prediction" found in the fifth chapter of the *'Tantra which Comprises the Supreme Path of the Means which Clearly Reveal All-Positive Pristine Cognition'* (Wylie: kun bzang ye shes gsal bar ston pa'i thabs kyi lam mchog 'dus pa'i rgyud, *Nyingma Gyubum* Vol.3) which Dudjom, *et al.*, render in English thus:

The Mahayoga tantras will fall onto the palace of King Ja. The Anuyoga tantras will emerge in the forests of Singhala [Dudjom *et al.* identify Singhala as located in Ceylon].

View

The particular view of Anuyoga is to realise the essence of the 'Threefold Maṇḍala of Samantabhadra' (Wylie: *kun tu bzang po dkyil 'khor gsum*):

1. "empty basic space" (Wylie: *skyes med pa'i dbyings*): the 'Primordial Maṇḍala of Samantabhadrī' (Wylie: *ye ji bzhin pa'i dkyil 'khor*).
2. "wisdom" (Wylie: *Ye shes*): the 'Natural Maṇḍala of Spontaneous Presence'(Wylie: *rang bzhin lhun grub kyi dkyil 'khor*).
3. "union of emptiness and wisdom" (Wylie: *chos kyi dbyings kyi ye shes*): the 'fundamental Maṇḍala of Enlightenment' (Wylie: *byang chub sems kyi dkyil 'khor*).

Stated differently:

The three mandalas of: Kuntuzangmo, the unborn dharmadhatu (dByings skye med kun tu bzang mo'i dkyil 'khor); whose unobstructed skillful means of luminosity is the mandala of Kuntuzangpo, the yeshe wisdom (Ye.shes kun tu.bzang po'i dkyil 'khor); and their inseparable union is the mandala of Great Bliss their son (Sras bde ba chen po'i dkyil 'khor).

Texts

Anuyoga is the middle category of the inner Tantras for the Nyingma school. This doxographical category, often called 'mdo' (Wylie; Sanskrit: *sūtra*; English: 'thread', 'continuity'), is not to be confused with the non-Tantric category by the same name. It contains several works that designate themselves as sūtras, as well as the important text "Compendium of the Buddhas' Intentionality" (Sanskrit: *Sarvatathagata svabhabhi sasa tantra*, Wylie: *sangs rgyas dgongs 'dus*) or Compendium of the Intentions (Wylie: dgongs pa 'dus pa'i mdo). This text which may or may not have ever existed in India; according to the colpohon it was translated from the language of Gilgit (*bru sha*), from whence all of the Anuyoga texts are said to have been brought to Tibet.

Altogether, there are three volumes of Anuyoga tantras amounting to nearly three thousand pages of Tibetan text. Although the mTshams brag edition of The Collected Tantras does not rigorously organise its texts according to sub-categories, the Anuyoga category may be further subdivided according to the following scheme from Dudjom Rinpoche (Dudjom, *et al.* 1991: p. 289) which varies from the earlier catalogues canonised by Jigme Lingpa and that of Dampa Deshegs:

1. The four root sutras (Wylie: *rtsa ba'i rgyud bzhi*).
2. The six tantras clarifying the six limits (Wylie: *mtha' drug gsal bar byed pa'i rgyud drug*).
3. The twelve rare tantras (Wylie: *dkon rgyud bcu gnyis*).
4. The Seventy Literary Scriptures (Wylie: *lung gi yi ge bdun cu*).

The Four Root Sutras (Wylie: Rtsa Ba'i Mdo Bzhi)

- Compendium of the Buddhas' Intentionality (Sanskrit: *Sarvatatathagata svabhabhi sasa tantra*, Wylie: *sangs rgyas dgongs 'dus*) or Compendium of the Intentions (Wylie: *dgongs pa 'dus pa'i mdo*).
- Knowing of All the Gathered (Wylie: *kun 'dus rig pa'i mdo*).
- Play of the Charnel Ground Cuckoo (Wylie: *dur khrod khu byug rol ba*).
- Majestic Wisdom's Wheel of Lightning (Wylie: *ye shes rngam pa klog gi 'khor lo*).

The Six Tantras Clarifying the Six Limits (Wylie: Mtha' Drug Gsal Bar Byed Pa'i Rgyud Drug)

- kun tu bzang po che ba rang la gnas pa'i rgyud.
- dbang bskur rgyal po.
- ting 'dzin mchog.
- skabs sbyor bdun pa.
- brtson pa don bden.
- dam tshig bkod pa.

The Twelve Rare Tantras (Wylie: Dkon Rgyud Bcu Gnyis)

- zhi ba lha rgyud.
- chos nyid zhi ba'i lha rgyud.
- khro bo'i lha rgyud chen mo.
- khro bo'i lha rgyud rtogs pa chen po.
- thugs rje chen po'i gtor rgyud (terminating colophon of the *Catalogue of the Rig 'dzin Tshe dbang nor bu rNying ma'i rgyud 'bum*.
- rnal 'byor gsang ba'i tshogs rgyud chen po.

- dpal 'bar khro mo.
- rak ta dmar gyi rgyud.
- me lha zhi bar gyur ba 'bar ba'i rgyud.
- khro bo'i sbyin bsregs rdo rje'i dur mo.
- hum mdzad chen mo.
- zla gsang chen mo.

The Seventy Literary Scriptures (Wylie: Lung Gi Yi Ge Bdun Cu)

This list remains to be enumerated.

Mindstream

The 'mind-stream doctrine' (Sanskrit: *citta santana*; Wylie: *thugs rgyud*; *sems rgyud*) is a union of the 'Mind Cycle' (Wylie: *sems sde*) of Atiyoga and Anuyoga proper and is reinforced by the *Guhyagarbha Tantra* literature and the *Kulayarāja Tantra* which comprised a major part of the transmitted precepts of the 'Zur Lineage' (Wylie: *zur lugs*):

This family was responsible for first formulating the transmitted precepts as such. In doing so, they made the *Compendium Sūtra* a major part of their system, placing it alongside the *Guhyagarbha Tantra* and the *kun byed rgyal po* to make their famous "sūtra-tantra-mind triad" (*mdo rgyud sems gsum*). These three works became the chief canonical texts of the Zur's transmitted precepts, corresponding to the respective doxographical classes of Anuyoga, Mahāyoga, and the Mind Class of Atiyoga (*sems sde*).

Mahayoga

Mahāyoga (Skt. "great yoga") is the designation of the first of the three Inner Tantras according to the ninefold division of practice used by the Nyingma school of Tibetan Buddhism.

Mahāyoga is held to emphasize the generation stage (or "development stage") of Tantra, where the succeeding two yana, anuyoga and atiyoga, emphasise the completion stage and the synthesis or transcendence of the two, respectively.

Practice

Reginald Ray (2002: p. 124) associates the Mahāyoga with removing the obscuration of aggression (or anger). The relative aspect of the two truths is mentioned and an embedded quotation by Tulku Thondup:

Mahāyoga-yana is associated with the masculine principle and is for those whose primary defilement is aggression. In Mahāyoga, one visualizes oneself as the divinity with consort. "All manifestation, thoughts and appearances are considered to be the sacred aspects of the divinities within relative truth," in the words of Tulku Thondup. By visualizing all phenomena as the deities of the mandala of buddhahood, in the development stage, all appearances are purified.

Ray (2002: p. 124) highlights the pre-eminent usage of visualization amongst the techniques of tantric sadhana and the teaching of the "eight cosmic commands":

One particular keynote of mahāyoga-yana has to do with the use of visualization. In the Vajrayana in general, one visualizes oneself as the buddha, thus giving external form to the enlightenment within. Like-wise, one visualizes the external world as pure and sacred, thus under-cutting the usual practice of taking things as impure and defiled. In mahāyoga, one comes to the realization that actually all of our everyday experience is a visualization. Just as we can visualize ourselves as a buddha and the world as pure, so we can visualize ourselves as an existent ego and the world as defiled. Realizing that all of our images and conceptions of reality are in fact complex visualizations, we gain a unique entry into the underpinnings of the conventional world and gain a certain kind of unparalleled leverage over it. This is reflected in the mahāyoga-yana teaching of the "eight cosmic commands," eight kinds of ways to intervene in the operation of the conventional world and alter its momentum for the benefit of others.

Mahāyoga Textual Tradition

As with the other yanas, Mahāyoga represents both a scriptural division as well as a specific emphasis of both view (Tibetan: *ta-ba*) and practice (Tibetan: *yod-pa*). Mahāyoga scriptures are further divided into two sections: the Sadhana section, consisting of practice texts for meditation on specific deities, and the Tantra section.

In introducing the *mTshams brag Edition of the Collected Tantras of the Ancients rnying ma rgyud 'bum*, the textual tradition of the Mahāyoga-yana, the "Tibetan and Himalayan Library" states:

The Mahāyoga section of the Collected Tantras of the Ancients is the largest of the three. It is divided into two major sections: the Tantra Series (*rgyud sde*) and the Practice Series (*sgrub sde*). One of the seminal Tantras of the Ancients found in this section is the Secret Essence Tantra or *gsang ba'i snying po'i rgyud*, which has spawned not only a plethora of Indo-Tibetan commentaries but also a heated debate in Tibet over its authenticity.

The "Tibetan and Himalayan Library" states that "although the *mTshams brag* edition of The Collected Tantras does not rigorously organize its texts according to sub-categories, the Mahāyoga category can be further subdivided according to the following scheme":

1. Tantra Series (*rgyud sde*)
    1. The eightfold set of root Magical Emanation Tantras (*Mayajala, rtsa bar gyur sgyu 'phrul sde brgyad*).
    2. The eighteenfold set of explanatory tantras (*bshad pa dang cha mthun gyi rgyud tantra sde bco brgyad*).
        1. Enlightened Body (*sku*).
        2. Enlightened Speech (*gsung*).
        3. Enlightened Mind (*thugs*).

4. Enlightened Qualities (*yon tan*).
5. Enlightened Activities (*phrin las*).

3. Miscellaneous.

2. Practice Series of the Eight Proclamation Deities (*sgrub sde bka' brgyad*).
   1. The Practice Series (*sgrub sde*).
      1. Summary of the Highest Intention (*bla ma dgongs pa 'dus pa*).
      2. Consortium of Sugatas (*bde gshegs 'dus pa*).
      3. Miscellaneous.
   2. The Eight Proclamation Deities (*bka' brgyad*).
      1. The Mañjushrī Cycle on Enlightened Form (*'jam dpal sku'i skor*).
      2. The Lotus Tantras on Enlightened Communication (*pad ma gsung gi rgyud*).
      3. The Real Tantras on Enlightened Mind (*yang dag thugs kyi rgyud*).
      4. The Nectar Tantras on Enlightened Qualities (*bdud rtsi yon tan gyi rgyud*).
      5. The Sacred Dagger Cycle on Enlightened Activities (*phrin las phur pa'i skor*).
      6. The Cycle on Invoking the Fierce Ma-mo Deities (*ma mo rbod gtong skor*).
      7. Offerings and Praises to Protect the Teachings (*bstan srung mchod bstod*).
      8. The Cycle on Fierce Mantras (*drag sngags skor*).
      9. Miscellaneous.
   3. Miscellaneous.
3. Miscellaneous.

Eighteen Great Tantras of Mahāyoga

The 'eighteen great tantras' (Wylie: *bshad pa dang cha mthun gyi rgyud tantra sde bco brgyad*) from the Tantra series described above are at the heart of the Mahāyoga tradition. These are grouped into 'five root tantras' (Wylie: *rtsa ba sku gsung thugs yon tan phrin las kyi rgyud chen po lnga*), 'five practice tantras' (Wylie: *sgrub pa lag len du bstan pa rol pa' rgyud chen po lnga*), and 'five activity tantras' (Wylie: *spyod pa'i yan lag tu 'gro ba'i rgyud chen po lnga*), and the 'two supplementary tantras' (Wylie: *ma tshang kha bskong ba'i rgyud chen po gnyis*). Together they are known as the *Māyājāla*. They are as follows:

The "Guhyagarbha Tantra" (Wylie: *rDo rje sems dpa' sgyu 'phrul drwa ba; gSang ba snying po*) is the foremost of all of these and it abridges the content of the seventeen others as follows:

Root Tantras

- Equalizing Buddhahood (the tantra of the body) (Wylie: *Sangs rgyas mnyam sbyor gyi rtsa ba mkha' 'gro ma bde mchog rtsa ba'i rgyud*).
- The Secret Moon, (the tantra of speech) (Wylie: *dPal Zla gsang thig le rtsa ba'i rgyud*).
- The Assembly of Secrets (Guhyasamāja Tantra) (the tantra of mind) (Wylie: *dPal gSang ba 'dus pa*).
- The Glorious Supreme Primal Tantra (the tantra of qualities) (Wylie: *dPal mchog dang po*).
- The Activity Garland Tantra (the tantra of activities) (Wylie: *Kar ma ma le*).

Practice Tantras

- The Heruka Practice Tantra (Wylie: *He ru ka rol pa'i rgyud*).
- The Hayagriva Supreme Practice Tantra (Wylie: *rTa mchog rol pa'i rgyud*).
- The Compassion Tantra (Wylie: *sNying rje rol pa'i rgyud*).
- The Nectar Practice Tantra (Wylie: *bDud rtsi rol pa'i rgyud*).
- The Arising of the Twelve Kilayas Tantra (Wylie: *Byit to ta ma rol pa'i rgyud; Phur pa bcu gnyis*).

Activity Tantras

- The Mountain Pile (Wylie: *Go 'phang dbang gis bgrod pa ri bo brtsegs pa'i rgyud*).
- The Awesome Wisdom Lightning (Wylie: *La spyod pas dor ba rngam pa glog gi 'khor lo'i rgyud*).
- The Array of Samayas (Wylie: *gZhi dam tshigs gis bzung ba bkod pa rgyal po'i rgyud*).
- The One-Pointed Samadhi (Wylie: *Nyams su ting 'dzin gyis blangs pa rtse gcig bsdus pa'i rgyud*).
- The Rampant Elephant (Wylie: *'Phang lta bas bcad pa glang po rab 'bog gi rgyud*).

Last Tantras that Complete Whatever is Incomplete

- The Vairochana Net of Magical Display (Wylie: *rNam par snang mdzad sgyu 'phrul drwa ba'i rgyud*).
- The Noble, Skilful Lasso, the Concise Lotus Garland (Wylie: *Thabs kyi zhags pa pad mo'i phreng ba'i rgyud*).

Eight Herukas of the Nyingma Mahāyoga

The eight Herukas (Wylie: *sgrub pa bka' brgyad*) of the Nyingma mahāyoga tradition (and their corresponding sadhanas) are said to have been received by Padmakara from the Eight Vidyadharas

(Tib. *Rigdzin*), or Eight Great Acharyas: Manjushrimitra, Nagarjuna, Vajrahumkara, Vimalamitra, Prabhahasti, Dhanasamskrita, Shintamgarbha and Guhyachandra. They were proficient in the practices of, respectively,

1) Yamantaka (Tib. *Jampal Shinje, 'jam dpal sku*) the wrathful Manjushri, the deity of body.

2) Hayagriva (Tib. *Pema Sung, padma gsung*) the wrathful Avalokiteshvara, the deity of speech.

3) Vishuddha/Sri Samyak (Tib. *Yangdak Thuk*, Wylie: *yang dag thugs*) the wrathful Vajrapani deity of mind.

4) Vajramrita (Tib. *Dudtsi Yonten, bdud rtsi yon tan*) the wrathful Samantabhadra, the deity of enlightened qualities.

5) Vajrakilaya/Vajrakumara (Tib. *Dorje Phurba, phur ba 'phrin las*), the wrathful Nivaranavishkambin, the deity of action.

6) Matarah (Tib. *Mamo Botong, ma mo rbod gtong*) the wrathful Akasagarbha, the deity of calling and dispatching.

7) Lokastotrapuja-natha (Tib. *Jigten Chotod, 'jig rten mchod bstod*) the wrathful Ksitigarbha, the deity of worldly offering and praise.

8) Vajramantrabhiru (Tib. *Mopa Dragnak, mod pa drag sngags*) the wrathful Maitreya, the deity of wrathful mantras.

Sahaja Yoga

Sahaja Yoga is a spiritual technique founded by Nirmala Srivastava, more widely known as Shri Mataji Nirmala Devi or as "Mother" by her followers, who are called Sahaja yogis. According to the movement, Sahaja Yoga is the state of self-realization produced by kundalini awakening and is accompanied by the experience of thoughtless awareness or mental silence.

Sahaja Yoga is not only the name of the movement, but also the technique the movement teaches and the state of awareness achieved by the technique. The movement teaches the belief that self-realization through kundalini awakening is a transformation which results in a more moral, united, integrated and balanced personality.

History

Sahaja Yoga started in India and England (where Nirmala Srivastava moved in 1974) and there are now Sahaja Yoga centres in almost 100 countries world-wide. Srivastava charged no money, insisting that her lesson was a birthright which should be freely available to all. "There can be no peace in the world until there is peace within," she said.

The word 'Sahaja' in Sanskrit has two components: saha meaning 'with' and ja meaning 'born'. *A Dictionary of Buddhism* gives the literal translation of Sahaja as "innate" and defines it as "denoting the natural presence of enlightenment (bodhi) or purity." and Yoga means *union* or *yoking* and refers to a spiritual path or a state of spiritual absorption. According to a book published by the movement, Sahaja Yoga means *spontaneous* and *born with you* meaning that the kundalini is born within us and can be awakened spontaneously, without effort.

The term 'Sahaja Yoga' goes back at least to the 15th Century Indian mystic Kabir. and has also been used to refer to Surat Shabd Yoga.

In 2000, the term 'Sahaja Yoga' was trademarked in the United States by Vishwa Nirmala Dharma.

Beliefs

Sahaja Yoga beliefs are seen by the organisation as a re-discovered ancient knowledge that should be treated respectfully and scientifically, like a hypothesis and if found by experiments as truth, should be accepted.Shri Mataji Nirmala Devi is considered to be an "avatar" by many of her followers and as a carrier of the divine presence which leads some critics to find the organization as cultic. Advanced concepts are not generally taught until a beginner is understood to have gained enough knowledge of their own subtle system through actual experience. Without direct experience of the meditation, some people have reported difficulties understanding or proceeding to the more advanced material. Sociologist, Judith Coney, for example, reported facing a challenge in getting behind what she called "the public facade". She described Sahaja yogis as adopting a low profile with uncommitted individuals to avoid unnecessary conflict.

Sahaja Yoga also states that spreading Sahaja Yoga techniques should be free for everyone.

Judith Coney observed that the movement tolerates a variety of world views and levels of commitment with some practitioners choosing to remain on the periphery.

The Subtle System – Chakras, Nadis and Void

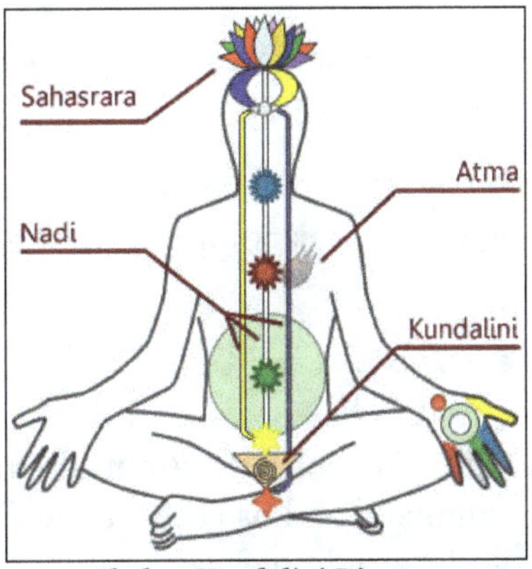

Chakra Kundalini Diagram.

Sahaja Yoga believes that in addition to our physical body there is a subtle body composed of nadis (channels) and chakras (energy centres). There is no biomedical evidence of chakras. Psychoanalyst Sudhir Kakar writes that Nirmala Srivastava's additions to this widespread traditional 'tantric' model include giving it a scientific, neurological veneer, an elaboration of the health aspects and an introduction of notions of traditional Christian morality. Nirmala Srivastava equates the Sushumna nadi with the parasympathetic nervous system, the Ida nadi with the left and the Pingala nadi with the right sides of the sympathetic nervous system.

Kundalini, Self-realization and Vibratory Awareness

Sahaja Yoga believes that the chakras can be balanced by awakening the kundalini in the sacrum bone, which is conceived of as a normally dormant 'mother' energy. Nirmala Srivastava has said that the kundalini is the reflection within us of the Holy Spirit or Adi (Primordial) Shakti. She has said that kundalini "is the desire of God.... and the desire of God is the Shakti" and that yoga is impossible without kundalini awakening. As the kundalini rises through these centres, the qualities of the chakras are said to begin manifesting spontaneously. Most illnesses are said to be a result of damage to the chakras, and kundalini is said to repair them.

According to Sahaja Yoga, once the sahasrara (topmost) chakra is pierced by the kundalini, a person will feel a cool breeze on top of their head and/or on their hands. The chakras and nadis are believed by Sahaja Yoga to have associated places on the hands. Sensations of heat or coolness in the hands, head and/or body are used to make purported diagnoses of imbalances in the different chakras and nadis. These sensations (referred to as 'vibrations') are interpreted in Sahaja Yoga as indicating Self-Realization or an "encounter with Reality." The vibrations sensed are believed to be an objective divine energy that can even be caught on camera.

A Sahaja Yoga belief is that upon self-realization, the practitioner may also experience thoughtless awareness (Nirvichar Samādhi).

Organization

Vishwa Nirmala Dharma (trans: Universal Pure Religion, also known as Sahaja Yoga International) is the organizational part of the movement. It is a registered organisation in countries such as Colombia, the United States of America, and Austria. It is registered as a religion in Spain.

The organisation is governed by the World Council for the Advancement of Sahaja Yoga (WCASY), proposed in 2003 and formed the following year.

In addition to directly promoting Sahaja Yoga, the council promotes Sahaja culture, runs schools, a health centre, a youth movement, and a project for the rehabilitation of "destitute women and orphaned children".

Schools

- The International Sahaja Public School in Dharamsala founded in 1990, teaches around 250 international students annually and has accepted children from the age of 6. India is said to be free from harmful Western influences, and children benefit from what is considered to be a more favourable environment.
- The Shri P.K.Salve Kala Pratishthan is an Indian Classical Music and Fine Arts academy that was founded in Vaitarna, India, in 2003.
- The Cabella Primary School in Italy was scheduled to open in September 2008, with the children attending the local village school in Rocchetta Ligure.
- An international kindergarten was opened in Borotin, Czech Republic.

- A small kindergarten and primary boarding school was opened in Canajoharie, New York in 2004. As of 2006 it had an enrolment of fourteen students from pre-kindergarten through grade 3.
- There has been a Sahaja Yoga school in Rome.

Yuvashakti

Sahaja Yoga's youth movement is called "Yuvashakti" (also "Nirmal Shakti Yuva Sangha"), from the Sanskrit words Yuva (Youth) and Shakti (Power).

The movement is active in forums such as the World Youth Conference and TakingITGlobal which aim at discussing global issues, and ways of solving them.

The Yuvashakti participated in the 2000 "Civil Society & Governance Project" in which they were "instrumental in reaching out to women from the poor communities and providing them with work".

Vishwa Nirmal Prem Ashram

The *Vishwa Nirmala Prem Ashram* is a not-for profit project by the NGO Vishwa Nirmala Dharma (Sahaja Yoga International) located in Noida, Delhi, India, opened in 2003. The ashram is a "facility where women and girls are rehabilitated by being taught meditation and other skills that help them overcome trauma".

Funding

The methods for practising Sahaja Yoga are made available free of charge to those interested. According to the official Sahaja Yoga website there is a fee for attending international pujas to cover costs and voluntary dakshina.

According to author David V. Barrett, "Shri Mataji neither charged for her lectures nor for her ability to give Self Realization, nor does one have to become a member of this organisation. She insisted that one cannot pay for enlightenment and she continued to denounce the false self-proclaimed 'gurus' who are more interested in the seekers' purse than their spiritual ascent". However, the movement had been criticised because of encouragement of its members to make donations to pay the travel charges for Mataji's visits to their respective countries.

Cult Allegations and Refutations

Judith Coney found that most people who leave the movement voluntarily, still had positive things to say about it, and described a discussion she attended regarding the level of secrecy within the group in which Sahaja yogis discussed the ways in which some of their beliefs were disguised when in contact with non-members as "frank and revealing". A smaller group of ex-members have made complaints against the movement which have been reported in the press. In 2001, *The Independent* reported that certain ex-members say "that Sahaja Yoga is a cult which aims to control the minds of its members". In 2005, *The Record* reported that some critics who feel that the group is a cult have started their own websites.

A 2008 court case in Brussels ruled that Sahaja Yoga had been wrongly labelled as a cult by a Belgian state authority and awarded the group compensation.

In 2013, *De Morgen* reported that the Belgian Department of State Security monitors how often politicians are contacted and lobbied by organisations. The list of organisations includes Sahaja Yoga, as well as Scientology and The Muslim Brotherhood.

In 2001, The *Evening Standard* reported that Sahaja Yoga has been "described as a dangerous cult" and "has a dissident website created by former members". The reporter, John Crace, wrote about an event he attended and noted that a Sahaja Yoga representative asked him to feel free to talk to whomever he wanted. He remarked, "Either their openness is a PR charm offensive, or they genuinely have nothing to hide." He proposed that "one of the key definitions of a cult is the rigour with which it strives to recruit new members" and concluded that there was no aggressive recruitment squeeze.

A 2001 INFORM leaflet says that the emphasis on complete devotion has led to problems and controversy. There is a culture amongst a minority of Sahaja yogis to believe that those who deviate in particular ways may be possessed by 'negativity' or may be said to be mentally abnormal. Those who fight the pressure to follow the Guru's suggestions and radically change their lifestyle risk being expelled. It is claimed that this may bring problems for those who still believe in the power of the Guru and fear 'losing vibrations'. This expulsion is not enforced but is something understood socially and other yogis are not expected to change the way they react to those who have been expelled. It is also not a permanent expulsion; there have been cases of returning Sahaja yogis following brief periods 'out'.

David V. Barrett wrote that some former members say that they were expelled from the movement because they "resisted influence that Mataji had over their lives". According to Barrett, the movement's founder's degree of control over members' lives has given rise to concerns. The Austrian Ministry for Environment, Youth and Family states that "Sahaja Yoga" regards Nirmala Srivastava as an authority who cannot be questioned.

Asana

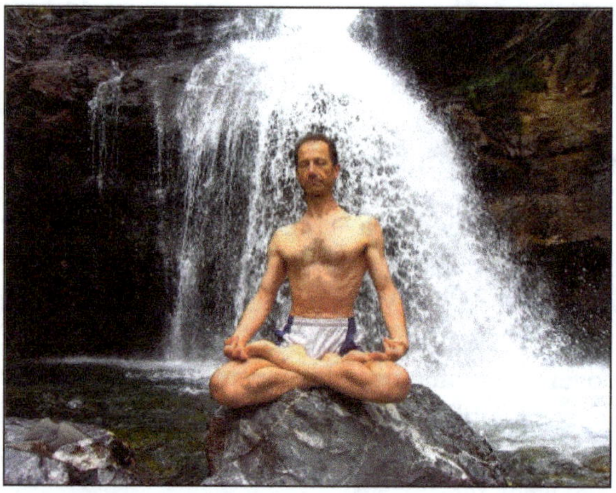

Padmasana or Lotus pose.

In yoga, asana refers both to the place in which a practitioner (*yogi* if male, *yogini* if female) sits and the posture in which he or she sits. In the Yoga Sutras, Patanjali defines "asana" as "to be seated in a position that is firm, but relaxed". Patanjali mentions the ability to sit for extended periods as one of the eight limbs of his system, known as ashtanga yoga.

Asanas are also performed as physical exercise where they are sometimes referred to as "yoga postures" or "yoga positions". Some asanas are arguably performed by many practitioners just for health purposes. Asanas do promote good health, although in different ways compared to physical exercises, "placing the physical body in positions that cultivate also awareness, relaxation and concentration".

Terminology

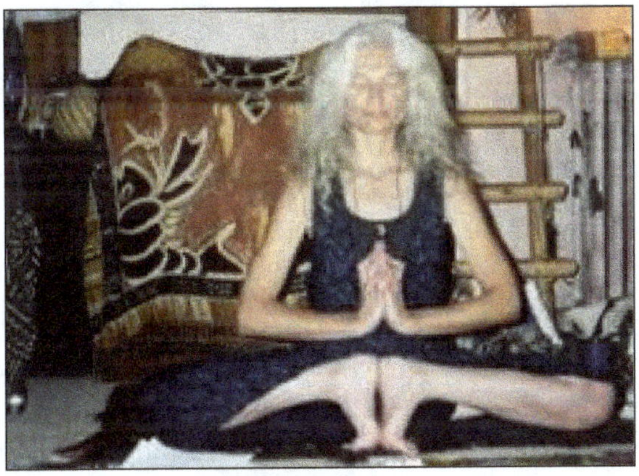

Mudra and Asana.

Asana Sanskrit: **आसन** *āsana* 'sitting down', < **आस** *ās* 'to sit down') originally meant a sitting position. The word *asana* in Sanskrit does appear in many contexts denoting a static physical position, although traditional usage is specific to the practice of yoga. Traditional usage defines asana as both singular and plural. In English, plural for asana is defined as asanas. In addition, English usage within the context of yoga practice sometimes specifies *yogasana* or *yoga asana*, particularly with regard to the system of the Ashtanga Vinyasa Yoga. However, *yogasana* is also the name of a particular posture that is not specifically associated with the Vinyasa system, and that while "ashtanga" (small 'a') refers to the eight limbs of Yoga delineated below, Ashtanga (capital 'A') refers to the specific system of Yoga developed by Sri Krishnamacharya at the Mysore Palace.

Yoga first originated in India. In the Yoga Sutras, Patanjali describes asana as the third of the eight limbs of classical, or Raja Yoga. Asanas are the physical movements of yoga practice and, in combination with pranayama or breathing techniques, constitute the style of yoga referred to as Hatha Yoga. In the Yoga Sutra, Patanjali describes asana as a "steady and comfortable posture", referring specifically to the seated, meditative postures used for meditation practices. He further suggests that meditation is the path to samādhi; transpersonal self-realization.

The eight limbs are, in order, the yamas (codes of social conduct), niyamas (self-observances), asanas (postures), pranayama (breath work), pratyahara (sense withdrawal or non-attachment), dharana (concentration), dhyana (meditation), and samadhi (realization of the true Self or Atman, and unity with Brahman (The Hindu Concept of Ultimate Reality)).

Common Practices

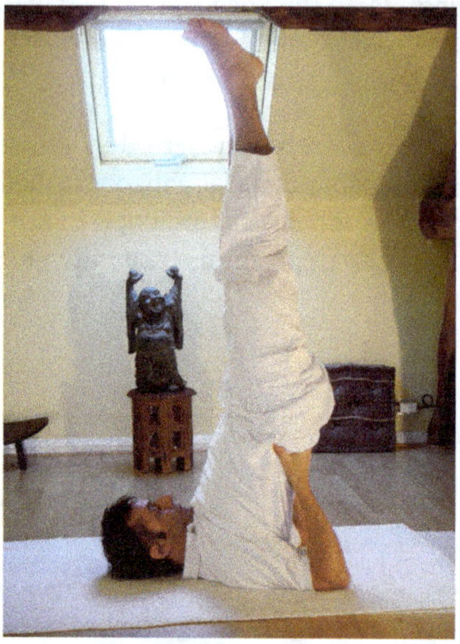

Sarvangasana.

In the Yoga Sutras, the only rule Patanjali suggests for practicing asana is that it be "steady and comfortable". The body is held poised with the practitioner experiencing no discomfort. When control of the body is mastered, practitioners are believed to free themselves from the duality of heat/cold, hunger/satiety, joy/grief, which is the first step toward the unattachment that relieves suffering.

Listed below are traditional rules for performing asanas:

- The stomach should be empty.
- Force or pressure should not be used, and the body should not tremble.
- Lower the head and other parts of the body slowly; in particular, raised heels should be lowered slowly.
- The breathing should be controlled. The benefits of asanas increase if the specific pranayama to the yoga type is performed.
- If the body is stressed, perform Corpse Pose or Child Pose
- Such asanas as Sukhasana or Shavasana help to reduce headaches.

Pranayama

Pranayama, or breath control, is the Fourth Limb of ashtanga, as set out by Patanjali in the Yoga Sutra. The practice is an integral part of both Hatha Yoga and Ashtanga Vinyasa Yoga but while performing asanas. They are to be practiced and perfected as individual practices of their own.

Patanjali discusses his specific approach to pranayama in verses 2.49 through 2.51, and devotes verses 2.52 and 2.53 of the Sutra to explaining the benefits of the practice. Patanjali describes pranayama as the control of the enhanced "life force" that is a result of practicing the various breathing techniques, rather than the exercises themselves. The entirety of breathing practices includes those classified as pranayama, as well as others called *svarodaya*, or the "science of breath". It is a vast practice that goes far beyond the limits of pranayama as applied to asana.

Surya Namaskara

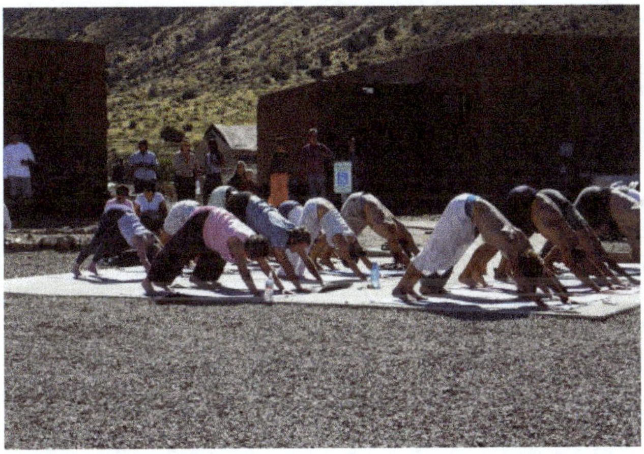

Adho Mukha Svanasana is the 5th and 8th asana in Sun Salutation.

Surya Namaskara, or the Salutation of the Sun, which is very commonly practiced in most forms of yoga, originally evolved as a type of worship of Surya, the Vedic solar deity, by concentrating on the Sun for vitalization. The practice supports development of the koshas, or temporal sheaths, of the subtle body.

The physical aspect of the practice 'links together' twelve asanas in a dynamically expressed series. A full round of Surya namaskara is considered to be two sets of the twelve asanas, with a change in the second set where the opposing leg is moved first. The asanas included in the sun salutation differ from tradition to tradition.

Benefits

The physical aspect of what is called yoga in recent years, the asanas, has been much popularized in the West due to the vast amount of benefits. Physically, the practice of asanas is considered to:

- improve flexibility.
- improve strength.
- improve balance.
- reduce stress and anxiety.
- reduce symptoms of lower back pain.
- be beneficial for asthma and chronic obstructive pulmonary disease (COPD).
- increase energy and decrease fatigue.

- shorten labor and improve birth outcomes.
- improve physical health and quality of life measures in the elderly.
- improve diabetes management.
- reduce sleep disturbances.
- reduce hypertension.
- improve blood circulation.
- reduce weight.

The emphasis on the physical benefits of yoga, attributed to practice of the asanas, has de-emphasized the other traditional purposes of yoga which are to facilitate the flow of prana (vital energy) and to aid in balancing the koshas (sheaths) of the physical and metaphysical body.

Number of Positions

In 1959, Swami Vishnu-devananda published a compilation of 66 basic postures and 136 variations of those postures. In 1975, Sri Dharma Mittra suggested that "there are an infinite number of asanas.", when he first began to catalogue the number of asanas in the *Master Yoga Chart of 908 Postures*, as an offering of devotion to his guru Swami *Kailashananda Maharaj*. He eventually compiled a list of 1300 variations, derived from contemporary gurus, yogis, and ancient and contemporary texts. This work is considered one of the primary references for asanas in the field of yoga today. His work is often mentioned in contemporary references for Iyengar Yoga, Ashtanga Vinyasa Yoga, Sivananda Yoga, and other classical and contemporary texts.

84 Classic Asanas

A group of 84 classic asanas taught by Lord Shiva is mentioned in several classic texts on yoga. Some of these asanas are considered highly important in the yogic canon: texts that do mention the 84 frequently single out the first four as necessary or vital to attain yogic perfection. However, a complete list of Shiva's asanas remains as yet unverified, with only one text attempting a complete corpus.

Patanjali's *Yoga Sutra* (4-2nd century BC) does not mention a single asana by name, merely specifying the characteristics of a good asana. Later yoga texts however, do mention the 84 Classic Asanas and associate them with Shiva.

The *Goraksha Samhita* (10-11th century CE), or *Goraksha Paddhathi*, an early hatha yogic text, describes the origin of the 84 classic asanas. Observing that there are as many postures as there are beings and asserting that there are 8,400,000 species in all, the text states that Lord Shiva fashioned an asana for each 100,000, thus giving 84 in all, although it mentions and describes only two in detail: the siddhasana and the padmasana.

The *Hatha Yoga Pradipika* (15th century CE) specifies that of these 84, the first four are important, namely the siddhasana, padmasana, bhadrasana and simhasana.

The *Hatha Ratnavali* (17th century CE) is one of the few texts to attempt a listing of all the 84, although 4 out of its list do not have meaningful translations from the Sanskrit, and 21 are merely mentioned without any description. In all, 52 asanas of the *Hatha Ratnavali* are confirmed and described by the text itself, or other asana corpora.

The *Gheranda Samhita* (late 17th century CE) asserts that Shiva taught 8,400,000 asanas, out of which 84 are preeminent, and "32 are useful in the world of mortals." These 32 are: siddhasana, padmasana, bhadrasana, muktasana, vajrasana, svastikasana, simhasana, gomukhasana, virasana, dhanurasana, mritasana, guptasana, matsyasana, matsyendrasana, gorakshana, paschimottanasana, utkatasana, sankatasana, mayurasana, kukkutasana, kurmasana, uttanakurmakasana, uttanamandukasana, vrikshasana, mandukasana, garudasana, vrishasana, shalabhasana, makarasana, ushtrasana, bhujangasana, and yogasana.

In *Shiva Samhita* (17–18th century CE) the poses ugrasana and svastikasana replace the latter two of the *Hatha Yoga Pradipika*.

Patenting

In 2007, public awareness of increasing attempts to patent traditional asanas in the US like for example the attempt made by Kolkata born, US based Yoga teacher Bikram Choudhury, and others, amounting to 130 yoga-related patents in the US documented that year, prompted the government of India to seek clarification on the guidelines for patenting asanas from the US Patent Office. In 2008, to clearly show that all asanas are public knowledge and therefore not patentable, the government of India formed a team of yoga gurus, government officials, and 200 scientists from the Council of Scientific and Industrial Research (CSIR) to register all known asanas in a public database. The team collected asanas from 35 ancient texts including the Hindu epics, the Mahabharata, the Bhagwad Gita, and Patanjali's Yoga Sutras and as of 2010, has identified 900 asanas for the database which was named the Traditional Knowledge Digital Library and made available to patent examiners.

Profiteering from Yoga

In contrast to the tradition that valued giving knowledge to students without commercial interests, yoga asana training in many regions has become a commercial venture. This has led to a deterioration in the standards of practice, and the practice has attracted criticisms such as being termed a 'body show'. There is a growing realization that Asanas is only one aspect of the practices prescribed in the yogic tradition.

Mudra

A mudra is a symbolic or ritual gesture in Hinduism and Buddhism. While some mudras involve the entire body, most are performed with the hands and fingers. A mudrā is a spiritual gesture and an energetic seal of authenticity employed in the iconography and spiritual practice of Indian religions.

One hundred and eight mudras are used in regular Tantric rituals.

In yoga, mudras are used in conjunction with pranayama (yogic breathing exercises), generally while seated in Padmasana, Sukhasana or Vajrasana pose, to stimulate different parts of the body involved with breathing and to affect the flow of prana in the body.

Nomenclature

The Chinese translation is *yin* (Chinese: 印; pinyin: *yìn*) or *yinxiang* (Chinese: 印相; pinyin: *yìnxiàng*). The Japanese and Korean pronunciation is "*in*".

Iconography

Mudra is used in the iconography of Hindu and Buddhist art of the Indian subcontinent and described in the scriptures, such as Nāṭyaśāstra, which lists 24 *asaṁyuta* ("separated", meaning "one-hand") and 13 *saṁyuta* ("joined", meaning "two-hand") mudras. Mudra positions are usually formed by both the hand and the fingers. Along with *āsanas* ("seated postures"), they are employed statically in the meditation and dynamically in the Nāṭya practice of Hinduism.

Hindu and Buddhist iconography share some mudras. In some regions, for example in Laos and Thailand, these are distinct but share related iconographic conventions.

According to Jamgon Kongtrul in his commentary on the *Hevajra Tantra*, the ornaments of wrathful deities and witches made of human bones (Skt: aṣṭhimudrā; Wylie: *rus pa'i rgyanl phyag rgya*) are also known as mudra "seals".

Indian Classical Dance

In Indian classical dance, the term "Hasta Mudra" is used. The *Natya Shastra* describes 24 mudras, while the *Abhinaya Darpana* of Nandikeshvara gives 28. In all their forms of Indian classical dance the mudras are similar, though the names and uses vary. There are 28 (or 32) root mudras in Bharata Natyam, 24 in Kathakali and 20 in Odissi. These root mudras are combined in different ways, like one hand, two hands, arm movements, body and facial expressions. In Kathakali, which has the greatest number of combinations, the vocabulary adds up to c. 900. Sanyukta mudras use both hands and asanyukta mudras use one hand.

Yogic Mudras

The classical sources for the mudras in yoga are the *Gheranda Samhita* and the *Hatha Yoga Pradipika*. The Hatha Yoga Pradipika states the importance of mudras in yoga practice:

Therefore the goddess sleeping at the entrance of Brahma's door should be constantly aroused with all effort, by performing mudra thoroughly.

In the 20th and 21st centuries, the yoga teacher Satyananda Saraswati, founder of the Bihar School of Yoga, continued to emphasize the importance of mudras in his instructional text *Asana, Pranayama, Mudrā, Bandha.*

Basic Mudra: Chin Mudrā

The thumb and forefinger on each of the hands are joined, forming a zero. The rest of the fingers are extended. The hands are placed palms-up on the thighs or knees while sitting in vajrasana. This mudrā activates the diaphragm, making for deep "stomach-breathing" as the diaphragm pushes out the internal organs when it descends towards the pelvis on inhalation. Slow breathing in a 5-2-4-2 mentally counted rhythm (being; 5 the exhalation, 2 the breath retention and 4 the inhalation) causes prana flow in the pelvis and in the legs.

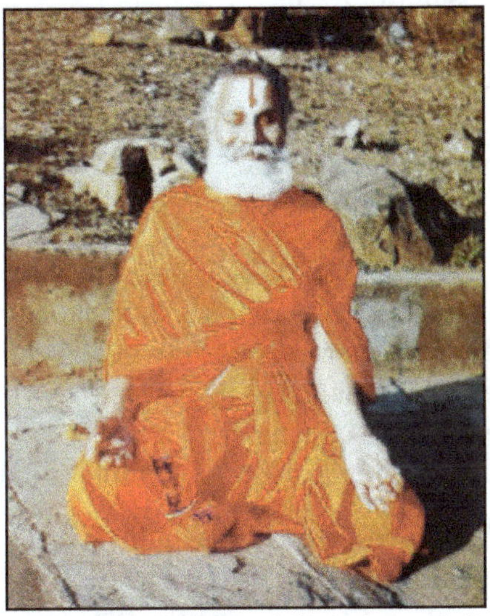

Rāmabhadrācārya meditating on the banks of the Mandakini River with fingers folded in the chin mudrā.

Basic Mudra: Chinmaya Mudrā

The thumb and forefinger are the same as in Chin Mudrā. The rest of the fingers are folded into a fist. The non-folded part of the forefinger and the middle finger should still be touching. As in Chin Mudrā, the hands are placed palms-up on the thighs while sitting in Vajrasana. This mudra activates the ribs, making them expand sideways on inhalation. Slow breathing in a 5-2-4-2 counted rhythm (being; 5 the exhalation, 2 the breath retention and 4 the inhalation) causes prana flow in the torso and in the throat.

Basic Mudra: Adi Mudrā

The thumb is folded into the palm, touching the base of the small finger. The rest of the fingers are folded over the thumb, to create a fist. The hands are placed palms-down on the thighs while sitting in Vajrasana. This mudra activates the pectoral muscles, making the chest expand forward on inhalation. Slow breathing in a 5-2-4-2 counted rhythm (being; 5 the exhalation, 2 the breath retention and 4 the inhalation) makes prana flow in the throat and in the head.

Basic Compact Mudra Brahma Mudrā

The hands are as in Adi Mudrā, but the palms face upwards and are located at the level of the navel, with the left and right knuckles and first finger joints touching. This is done while sitting in Vajrasana. Breathing becomes full: in inhalation, the diaphragm descends, the ribs then expand, and then the pectoral muscles move forward. Exhalation works in the same order, which creates a "wave" or ripple effect.

Advanced Compact Mudra: Prana Mudrā

A complicated mudra combining hand gestures, synchronized movement from gesture to gesture within the breath cycle, and meditation. The mudrā is practiced sitting in Siddhasana. Even a single breath cycle of this mudra can significantly stimulate the body. It is described in the book, Theories of the Chakras, by Hiroshi Motoyama.

Common Buddhist Mudrās

Abhaya Mudrā

Korea's National Treasure 119. The right hand shows abhaya mudra while the left is in the varada mudra.

The *Abhayamudra* "gesture of fearlessness" represents protection, peace, benevolence and the dispelling of fear. In Theravada Buddhism it is usually made while standing with the right arm bent and raised to shoulder height, the palm facing forward, the fingers closed, pointing upright and the left hand resting by the side. In Thailand and Laos, this mudra is associated with the walking Buddha, often shown having both hands making a double abhaya mudra that is uniform.

This mudra was probably used before the onset of Buddhism as a symbol of good intentions proposing friendship when approaching strangers. In Gandharan art, it is seen when showing the action of preaching. It was also used in China during the Wei and Sui eras of the 4th and 7th centuries.

This gesture was used by the Buddha when attacked by an elephant, subduing it as shown in several frescoes and scripts. In Mahayana Buddhism, the northern schools' deities often paired it with another mudra using the other hand.

Bhūmisparśa Mudrā

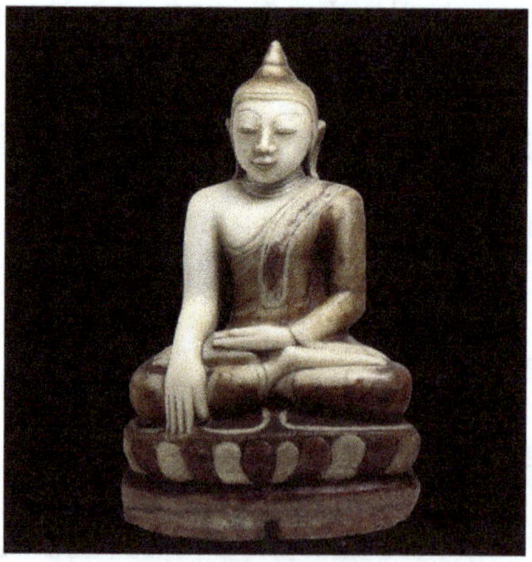

Buddha sitting in bhūmisparśa mudrā. Birmany. White marble with traces of polychromy. Gallo-Roman Museum of Lyon.

The *bhūmisparśa* or "earth witness" mudra of Gautama Buddha is one of the most common iconic images of Buddhism. It depicts the Buddha sitting in meditation with his left hand, palm upright, in his lap, and his right hand touching the earth. It represents the Buddha asking Pṛthivi, the devi of the earth, that she witness his enlightenment when he was threatened by demon king Mara.

Bodhyangi Mudrā

The *Bodhyangi mudrā*, the "mudrā of the six elements," or the "fist of wisdom," is a gesture entailing the left-hand index finger being grasped with the right hand. It is commonly seen on statues of the Vairocana Buddha.

Dharmachakra Mudrā

The Buddha preached his first sermon after his Enlightenment in Deer Park in Sarnath. The dharmachakra or "turning of the wheel" mudrā represents that moment. In general, only Gautama Buddha is shown making this mudrā except Maitreya as the dispenser of the Law. Dharmacakra mudrā is two hands close together in front of the chest in vitarka with the right palm forward and the left palm upward, sometimes facing the chest. There are several variants such as in the Ajanta Caves frescoes, where the two hands are separated and the fingers do not touch. In the Indo-Greek style of Gandhara, the clenched fist of the right hand seemingly overlies the fingers joined to the thumb on the left hand. In pictorials of Hōryū-ji in Japan the right hand is superimposed on the left. Certain figures of Amitābha, Japan are seen using this mudra before the 9th century.

Dhyāna Mudrā

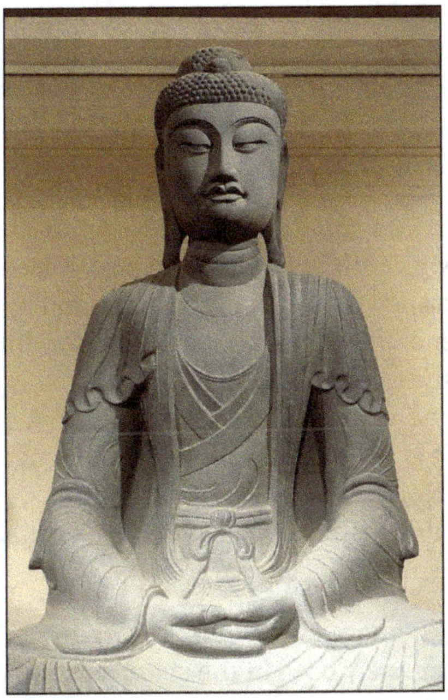

Amitābha statue in Hanoi, Vietnam, demonstrating dhyana mudra.

The *Dhyāna mudrā* ("meditation mudra") is the gesture of meditation, of the concentration of the Good Law and the saṅgha. The two hands are placed on the lap, right hand on left with fingers fully stretched (four fingers resting on each other and the thumbs facing upwards towards one another diagonally), palms facing upwards; in this manner, the hands and fingers form the shape of a triangle, which is symbolic of the spiritual fire or the Triratna (the three jewels). This mudra is used in representations of the Śākyamuni Buddha and Amitābha Buddha. Sometimes the Dhyāna mudrā is used in certain representations of Bhaiṣajyaguru as the Medicine Buddha, with a medicine bowl placed on the hands. It originated in India most likely in the Gandhāra and in China during the Wei period. This mudra was used long before the Buddha as yogis have used it during their concentration, healing, and meditation exercises.

It is heavily used in Southeast Asia in Theravāda Buddhism; however, the thumbs are placed against the palms. (Dhyāna mudrā is also known as *Samādhi mudrā* or *Yoga mudrā*; Japanese: *Jō-in, Jōkai Jō-in*; Chinese: *Ding Yin.*)

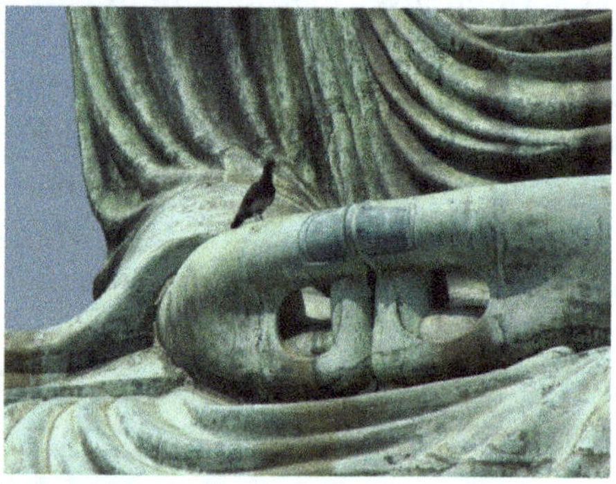

Hands of Amitābha statue at Kōtoku-in in Kamakura, demonstrating *mida no jōin*.

The *mida no jōin* (弥陀定印) is the Japanese name of a variation on the mudra, where the index fingers are brought together with the thumbs. This was predominately used in Japan in an effort to distinguish Amitābha (hence "mida" from Amida) from the Vairocana Buddha, and was rarely used elsewhere.

Varada Mudrā

The *Varada mudrā* "generosity gesture" signifies offering, welcome, charity, giving, compassion and sincerity. It is nearly always shown made with the left hand by a revered figure devoted to human salvation from greed, anger and delusion. It can be made with the arm crooked and the palm offered slightly turned up or in the case of the arm facing down the palm presented with the fingers upright or slightly bent. The Varada mudrā is rarely seen without another mudra used by the right hand, typically abhaya mudrā. It is often confused with vitarka mudrā, which it closely resembles. In China and Japan during the Northern Wei and Asuka periods, respectively, the fingers are stiff and then gradually begin to loosen as it developed over time, eventually leading to the Tang dynasty standard where the fingers are naturally curved.

In India, varada mudra is used in images of Avalokiteśvara from the Gupta Empire (4th and 5th centuries). Varada mudrā is extensively used in the statues of Southeast Asia.

Vajra Mudrā

The *Vajra mudrā* "thunder gesture" is the gesture of knowledge. An example of the application of the Vajra mudrā is the seventh technique (out of nine) of the *Nine Syllable Seals*.

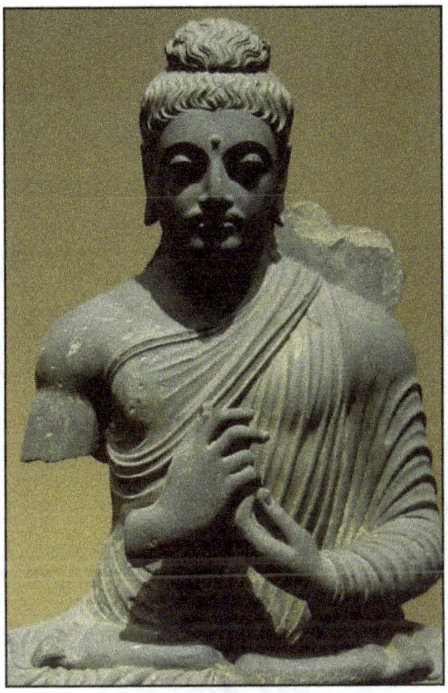

Vajra Mudrā.

Vitarka Mudrā

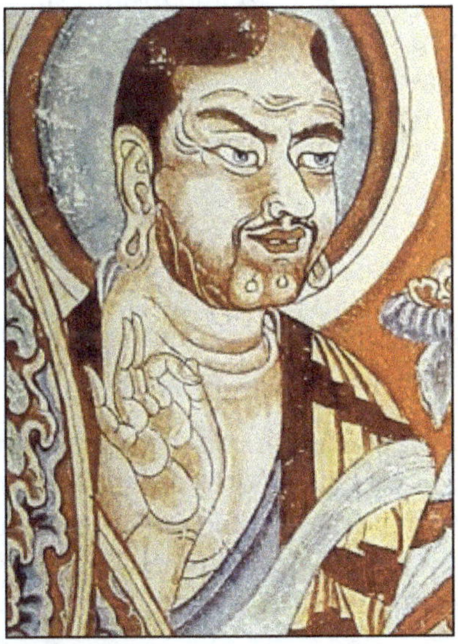

Vitarka mudrā, Tarim Basin, 9th century.

The *Vitarka mudrā* "mudra of discussion" is the gesture of discussion and transmission of Buddhist teaching. It is done by joining the tips of the thumb and the index together, and keeping the other fingers straight very much like the abhaya and varada mudrās but with the thumbs touching the index fingers. This mudra has a great number of variants in Mahayana Buddhism. In Tibetan Buddhism, it is the mystic gesture of Tārās and bodhisattvas with some differences by the deities in Yab-Yum. Vitarka mudrā is also known as *Prajñāliṅganabhinaya* and *Vyākhyāna mudrā* ("mudra of explanation").

Jñāna Mudrā

The *Jñāna mudrā* ("mudra of wisdom") is done by touching the tips of the thumb and the index together, forming a circle, and the hand is held with the palm inward toward the heart.

Karana Mudrā

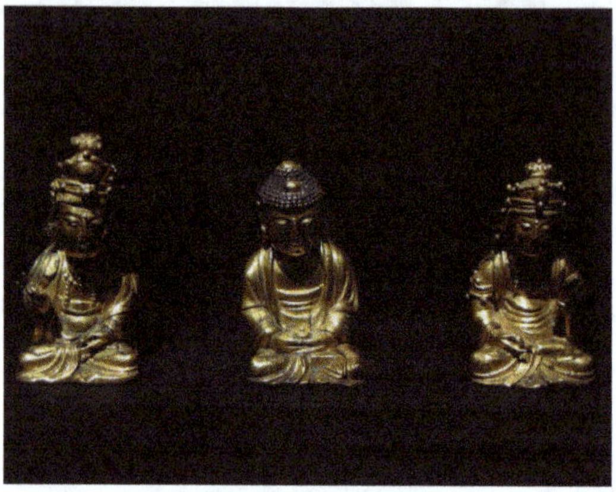

Joseon Dynasty figure on the left makes the Karana mudrā.

The *Karana mudrā* is the mudra which expels demons and removes obstacles such as sickness or negative thoughts. It is made by raising the index and the little finger, and folding the other fingers. It is nearly the same as the gesture known as corna in many 'western' countries, the difference is that in the Karana mudra the thumb does not hold down the middle and ring finger. (This mudra is also known as *Tarjanī mudrā*; Japanese: *Funnu-in, Fudō-in*).

Martial Arts and Mudra

Various Asian martial arts forms contain positions identical to these mudras.

Muromoto (2003) in discussing his experience of mudra in relation to his martial arts training makes reference to Mikkyō, Tendai and Shingon Buddhism:

One of the more curious things that I encountered in my martial arts training was the use of mudra in combative arts. Mudra (Japanese: in), for those who aren't familiar with them, are these weird hand gestures that are derived from esoteric Buddhism (mikkyo), particularly the Tendai and Shingon sects. These gestures are supposed to generate spiritual focus and power which then are manifested in some way externally.

Muromoto (2003) states a lineage of mudra in martial arts and evokes Koryū, Ryū, Kantō, Tenshin Shōden Katori Shintō-ryū, Risuke Ōtake and Donn F. Draeger:

In any case, I had known of the use of mudra in koryu ("old" martial arts) since the time I was privy to a discussion with the training master of the Tenshin Shoden Katori Shinto-ryu, Otake Risuke, and the late Donn F. Draeger. Otake sensei described some of the mudra used in his school, which is one of the oldest martial ryu still in existence in Kanto (Eastern) Japan.

In relation to charting a historical tributary to mudra within Japanese fighting culture, Muromoto

(2003) incorporates Shintō, Samurai, Tokugawa shogunate, Neo-Confucianism, Zen, the Kamakura shogunate, the Edo period, Takuan Sōhō and Hakuin Ekaku:

The use of mudra and other aspects of mikkyo are found in many instances in many koryu, because mikkyo and Shinto were the religions of the samurai who founded those ryu that were created before the 17th century. Subsequent ryu developed after the imposition of the Tokugawa government were heavily influenced by Neo-Confucianism, and then later by Zen Buddhism. Although Zen was popularized among the warrior class in the Kamakura period, the 14th century, it did not greatly affect martial arts until the latter part of the Edo Period, with the writings of the Zen priests Takuan and Hakuin. And even at that, Edo Period (1600-1868) martial arts were equally influenced by Neo-Confucianism and even, in the latter part, mystical Shinto.

Muromoto (2003) textually maps the execution of the knifehand strike mudrā:

Mikkyo uses mudra most often in combination with various rituals, chants and so on. One common mudra is that of the "knife hand," or shuto. The first two fingers are extended while the thumb and other fingers are clenched. If you look closely, you may see this movement subtly hidden in some koryu kata, especially by old schools such as the Tenshin Shoden Katori Shinto-ryu, or in statues of divine Buddhist beings. This represents the sword of enlightenment, which cuts away all delusions. Sometimes the tips of the extended fingers are grasped in the fist of the other hand. There is a symbolic meaning for this, derived from mikkyo.

Khecarī Mudrā

Khecarī Mudrā (Sanskrit, **खेचरी मुद्रा**) is a yoga practice which is carried out by placing the tongue above the soft palate and into the nasal cavity. In the beginning stages and applicable for most practitioners, the tip of the tongue touches the soft palate as far back as possible without straining or placed in contact with the uvula at the back of the mouth. Variant spellings include Khechari Mudra, Kecharimudra, and Kechari Mudra. *Mudrā* (Sanskrit, **मुद्रा**, literally "seal"), when used in yoga, is a position that is designed to awaken spiritual energies in the body.

The buddhist Pali canon contains three passages in which the Buddha describes pressing the tongue against the palate for the purposes of controlling hunger or the mind (example), depending on the passage. However, there is no mention of the tongue being inserted into the nasopharynx as in true kechari mudra.

A hathayoga text, the *Khecarīvidyā*, states that kechari mudra enables one to raise Kundalini and access various stores of amrita in the head, which subsequently flood the body. Siva, in the same text, gives instructions on how to cut the lingual frenulum as a necessary prerequisite for the kechari mudra practice.

A tantric Saiva text, the *Mālinīvijayottaratantra*, warns:

[If] his mouth fills with a slightly salty liquid that smells of iron then he should not drink it but spit it out. He should practice thus until [the liquid] becomes sweet-tasting.

Bhattacharyya defines Khecarī Mudrā as "name of Yogic posture which bestows spiritual attainment and enables one to overcome disease and death." He explains that "*Kha* denotes *brahman*, and that power which moves (*cara*) as the kinetic energy of *brahman* is known (as) Khecarī." Singh defines Khecarī Mudrā as "the bliss of the vast expanse of spiritual consciousness, also known as divya mudrā or Śivāvasthā (the state of Śivā)." He further identifies it in a higher sense—with the end state of consciousness, and not just the physical posture used to achieve that end: "So Khecarī Mudrā in Śaiva āgama means a state of universal consciousness which is the state of Śiva." Abhinavagupta, in his *Tantraloka*, states that all other mudras derive from Khecarī mudrā, which he describes as "the stance of moving or flying through the void of the supreme consciousness." The practice is also mentioned in the *Hatha Yoga Pradipika* (III. 6-7).

In recent times, it was taught by Paramahansa Yogananda as a part of Kriya Yoga practice. Yogananda stated that:

Through the performance of *Kechari Mudra*, touching the tip of the tongue to the uvula, or "little tongue," (or placing it in the nasal cavity behind the uvula), that divine life-current draws the *prana* from the senses into the spine and draws it up through the *chakras* to *Vaishvanara* (Universal Spirit), uniting the consciousness with spirit.

According to Swami Kriyananda, "The assumption of this mudra helps to hasten the advent of deep spiritual states of consciousness." Swami Sivananda described Khecarī Mudrā as "the best of all Mudras."

In Kriya Yoga, the benefits of Khecarī Mudrā are achieved by pronouncing certain vowel while breathing in and breathing out.

Kriyā

Kriyā (in Sanskrit "action, deed, effort" most commonly refers to a "completed action", technique or practice within a yoga discipline meant to achieve a specific result. Another meaning of Kriya is an outward physical manifestation of awakened kundalini, such as a spontaneous body movement related to Kundalini energy flow. *O KriyaShakti* is "a power of thought" said to be greatly studied by yogis.

Etymology

Kriyā is a Sanskrit term, derived from the Sanskrit root, *kri*, meaning "to do". *Kriyā* means "action, deed, effort". The word karma is also derived from the Sanskrit root √*kṛ* (kri) कृ, meaning "to do, make, perform, accomplish, cause, effect, prepare, undertake". Karma is related to verbal proto-Indo-European root *kwer- "to make, form".

The root *kṛ* (kri) is very common in ancient Sanskrit literature, and it is relied upon to explain ideas in Rigveda, other Vedas, Upanishads, Puranas, the Epics of Hinduism. The root "kri" also appears in the word Sanskrit, to imply a language that is "well made".

Origins

Bhagavad Gita

Kriya has been preserved in the *Bhagavad Gita*. According to Paramahansa Yogananda in his book *God Talks with Arjuna: The Bhagavad Gita*, Krishna refers to and describes Kriya Yoga:

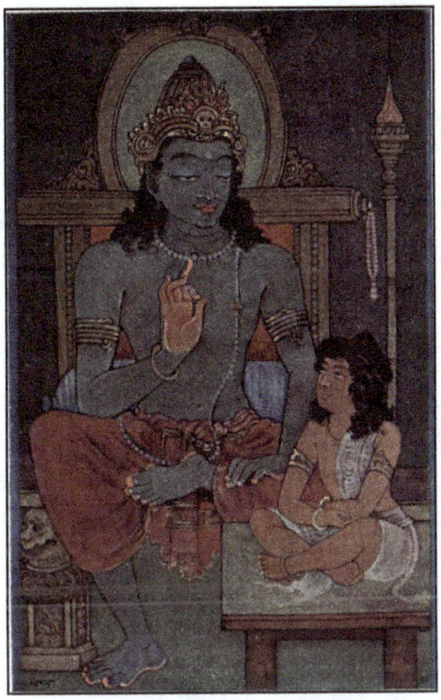

Krishna instructing Arjuna.

Offering inhaling breath into the outgoing breath, and offering the outgoing breath into the inhaling breath, the yogi neutralizes both these breaths; he thus releases the life force from the heart and brings it under his control.

Yoga Sutras of Patanjali

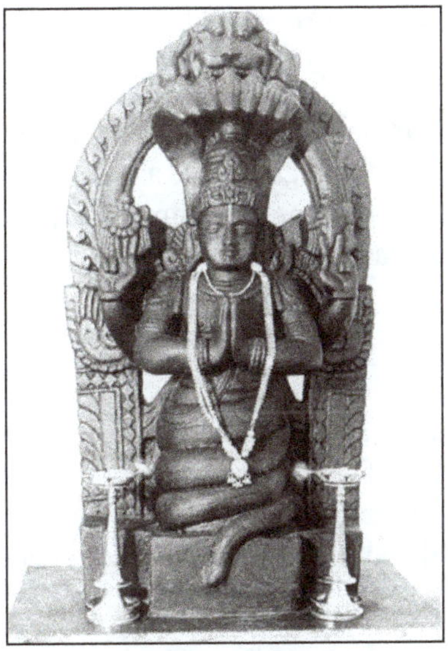

Patañjali statue (traditional form indicating Kundalini or incarnation of Shesha).

The *Yoga Sutras of Patanjali* are a composite of various texts. According to Feuerstein, the *Yoga Sutras* are a condensation of two different traditions, namely "eight limb yoga" (*ashtanga yoga*) and action yoga (*Kriyā yoga*), the description of the eight limbs being an interpolation into the text on *kriya*.

According to Hartranft and Govindan, Patanjali gives a description of Kriya Yoga in the second chapter. According to George Feuerstein, *kriya yoga* is contained in chapter 1, chapter 2 verse 1-27, chapter 3 except verse 54, and chapter 4. The "eight limb yoga" is described in chapter 2 verse 28-55, and chapter 3 verse 3 and 54.

According to Miller, *Kriya yoga* is the "active performance of yoga". It is part of niyama, "observances", the second limb of Patanjali's eight limbs. According to Miller, *Kriya yoga* is a threefold discipline, involving ascetic practice, the study and chanting of sacred hymns and syllables, and dedication to the Lord of Yoga.

Miller also notes that some commentators regard the first five limbs together as *kriya yoga*, but that Patanjali himself states *kriya yoga* to be a subset of the second limb. According to Mukunda Stiles, *Kriya Yoga* is defined in the first sutra of the second chapter:

Practice characterized by rigor and vigilance toward itself, without attachment to the outcome, is known as kriya yoga.

Contemporary usage

Mahavatar Babaji

The story of Lahiri Mahasaya receiving initiation into Kriya Yoga by the yogi Mahavatar Babaji in 1861 is recounted in *Autobiography of a Yogi*. Yogananda wrote that at that meeting, Mahavatar Babaji told Lahiri Mahasaya, "The Kriya Yoga that I am giving to the world through you in this nineteenth century, is a revival of the same science that Krishna gave millenniums ago to Arjuna; and was later known to Patanjali, and to Christ, St. John, St. Paul, and other disciples". Yogananda also wrote that Babaji and Christ were in continual communion and together, "have planned the spiritual technique of salvation for this age."

Yogananda was asked by Mahavatar Babaji to bring Kriya Yoga to the West. Through Lahiri Mahasaya to his disciple, Sriyukteswar to Yogananda, a disciple of Sriyukteswar Giri, Yogananda then brought Kriya Yoga to the United States and Europe beginning in 1920 and continues to this day through his organization Self-Realization Fellowship. In India the fellowship is called Yogoda Satsanga Society of India.

According to Yogananda,:

Kriya Yoga is a simple, psychological method by which human blood is decarbonated and recharged with oxygen. The atoms of this extra oxygen are transmuted into life current to rejuvenate the brain and spinal centers. By stopping the accumulation of venous blood, the yogi is able to lessen or prevent the decay of tissues. The advanced yogi transmutes his cells into energy.

Sudarshan Kriya

Sudarshan Kriya is a set of breathing techniques promoted since 1982 by Sri Sri Ravi Shankar, and is different from Kriya Yoga. Sudarshan Kriya is taught in various Art of Living programs.

According to the *Times of India*, Sudarshan Kriya works on mental, physical and spiritual levels.

Scientifically, Sudarshan Kriya improves antioxidant status at the enzyme and the gene level and reduce DNA damage and cell aging.

Sudharshan Kriya employs a variety of breathing patterns. Every emotion has breathing patterns; for example, if one gets angry then one's breath is short and fast. Similarly, breathing affects the mind (for example, a deep, long breath relaxes the mind.) Through breathing in different patterns, one can influence emotions and gain control over one's mind. Research suggested that it helps in improving well being (improving immunity and detoxification), and peace of mind (reduce stress, enhance brain function).

A research published in April 2013 observed that a comprehensive practice of Yoga, Sudarshan Kriya and Pranayam has rapid and significant effect on gene expression suggesting long term beneficial effects even at the molecular level.

Baba Haidakhan

Publications on Babaji describe Kriya Yoga as practiced by Baba Haidakhan who died in 1984. Haidakhan Babaji, simply called "Babaji" or Bhole Baba by his students and devotees, was a teacher who appeared in northern India (Uttarakhand) and taught publicly from 1970 to 1984.

Some modern teachers and institutions consider the entire Yoga Sutras to be Kriya Yoga, although Patanjali only relates the term Kriya Yoga to these three foundation practices (tapas, swadhyaya, Ishwara pranidhana). Breathing practices with attention along the spine are often included, along with other physical practices. It is useful for the student of yoga to be aware of these different approaches, so as to not get confused by the various public offerings.

Yamas

Yamas, and its complement, Niyamas, represent a series of "right living" or ethical rules within Hinduism and Yoga. They are a form of moral imperatives, commandments, rules or goals. The *Yamas* are the "don't do these" list of self-restraints, typically representing commitments that affect one's relations with others and self. The complementary Niyamas represent the "do these" list of observances, and together Yamas and Niyamas are personal obligations to live well.

The earliest mention of the word *Yamas* is in the Rigveda, and over fifty texts of Hinduism, from its various traditions, discuss Yamas. Patañjali lists five *yamas* in his Yoga Sūtras. Ten yamas are codified as "the restraints" in numerous Hindu texts including Yajnavalkya Smriti in verse 3.313, the Śāṇḍilya and Vārāha Upanishads, the *Hatha Yoga Pradipika* by Svātmārāma, and the Tirumantiram of Tirumular.

The most often mentioned Yamas are – Ahimsa (non-violence), Satya (non-falsehood, truthfulness), Asteya (non-stealing), Mitahara (non-excess in food, moderation in food), Kṣhamā (non-agitation about suffering, forgiveness), Dayā (non-prejudgment, compassion) are among the widely discussed Yamas. The Yamas apply broadly and include self-restraints in one's actions, words and thoughts.

Etymology and Meaning

The earliest mention of *Yamas* is found in the Hindu scripture Rigveda, such as in verse 5.61.2. The word in the Rigveda means a "rein, curb", the act of checking or curbing, restraining such as by a charioteer or a driver. The term evolves into a moral restraint and ethical duty in the Upanishads, the Dharmasutras, the Mahabharata and numerous later texts, where it means self-control, voluntary and inner-directed forbearance.

Yamas is the Sanskrit word for "restraint," states Stephen Sturgess, particularly "from actions, words, or thoughts that may cause harm".

Five Yamas

The five yamas listed by Patañjali in *Yogasūtra* 2.30 are:

1. Ahiṃsā (**अहिंसा**): Nonviolence, non-harming other living beings.
2. Satya (**सत्य**): truthfulness, non-falsehood.
3. Asteya (**अस्तेय**): non-stealing.
4. Brahmacharya (**ब्रह्मचर्य**): chastity, marital fidelity or sexual restraint.
5. Aparigraha (**अपरिग्रहः**): non-avarice, non-possessiveness.

Ten Yamas

The ten yamas listed by Śāṇḍilya Upanishad, as well as by Svātmārāma are:

1. Ahiṃsā (**अहिंसा**): Nonviolence.
2. Satya (**सत्य**): truthfulness.
3. Asteya (**अस्तेय**): not stealing.
4. Brahmacharya (**ब्रह्मचर्य**): chastity, marital fidelity or sexual restraint.
5. Kṣamā (**क्षमा**): forgiveness.
6. Dhṛti (**धृति**): fortitude.
7. Dayā (**दया**): compassion.
8. Ārjava (**आर्जव**): non-hypocrisy, sincerity.
9. Mitāhāra (**मितहार**): measured diet.
10. Śauca (**शौच**): purity, cleanliness.

Other Numbers of Yamas

At least sixty (60) ancient and medieval era Indian texts are known so far that discuss *Yamas*. Most are in Sanskrit, but some are in regional Indian languages. Of the sixty, the lists in eleven of these texts are similar, but not the same, as that of Patanjali's. Other texts list between 1 and 10 *Yamas*, however 10 is the most common.

The order of listed yamas, the names and nature of each yamas, as well as the relative emphasis vary between the texts. Some texts use the reverse of *Niyamas* in other texts, as Yamas; for example, *Vairagya* (dispassion from hedonism, somewhat reverse of the niyama *Tapas*) is described in verse 33 of Trishikhi Brahmana Upanishad in its list for Yamas. Many texts substitute one or more different concepts in their list of *Yamas*. For example, in the ten *Yamas* listed by Yatidharma Sangraha, Akrodha (non-anger) is included as a *Yamas*. Ahirbudhnya Samhita in verse 31.19 and Darshana Upanishad in verses 1.14-15 include *Dayā* as a Yamas, and explain it as the ethical restraint of not jumping to conclusions, being compassionate to every being and considering suffering of others as one's own. In verse 31.21, Ahirbudhnya Samhita includes K□hamā as the virtue of forgiveness and restraint from continued agitation from wrong others have done. Mahakala Samhita in verses II.11.723 through II.11.738 lists many of the 10 *Yamas* above, but explains why it is a virtue in a different way. For example, the text explains *Dayā* (or Dayaa) is an ethical precept and the restraint from too much and too little emotions. It suggests *Dayā* reflects one's inner state, is the expression of kindness towards kin, friend, stranger and even a hostile person, and that one must remain good and kind no matter what the circumstances. This view for the Yamas of *Dayā* is shared in Shandilya Upanishad and Jabala Darshana Upanishad. Atri Samhita in verse 48, lists *Anrshamsya* (**आनृशंस्य**) as the restraint from cruelty to any living being by one's actions, words or in thoughts. Shivayoga Dipika in verse 2.9 substitutes *Sunrta* for *Satya*, defining Sunrta as "sweet and true speech".

Ahimsa, Satya, Asteya, Mitahara, K□hamā, Dayā are among the widely discussed Yamas ethical concepts by majority of these texts.

Related Concepts

Yamas are related to Niyamas in ancient and medieval era Indian texts. The former are restraints (the "don'ts") of virtuous life, while the latter are observances (the "dos").

Some texts such as the Hatha Yoga Pradipika use the classification flexibly, where yamas (restraints, the "don'ts") are understood as reverse of niyamas (positive attitudes, behaviors, the "dos"). For example, *Ahimsa* and *Mitahara* are called as yama as well as niyama in verses 17 and 40 of Book 1. In verse 1.40, Hatha Yoga Pradipika calls *Ahimsa* (non-violence and non-injuring anyone by one's actions, words or in thoughts) as the highest virtuous habit, *Mitahara* (moderation in one's eating and drinking habits) as the best personal restraint, and Siddhasana as the foremost of Asanas.

Niyama

Niyama (Sanskrit: **नियम**) literally means positive duties or observances. In Indian traditions, particularly Yoga, *niyamas* and its complement, Yamas, are recommended activities and habits for healthy living, spiritual enlightenment and liberated state of existence. It has multiple meanings depending on context in Hinduism. In Buddhism, the term extends to the determinations of nature, as in the Buddhist *niyama dhammas*. In Pāli the spelling *niyāma* is often used.

Hinduism

Virtues are extensively discussed in various ancient and medieval era texts of Hinduism. In its Yoga school, they are described in first two of eight limbs (steps, branches, components). The first limb is called *yamas*, which include virtuous self-restraints (the "don'ts"). The second limb is called *niyamas* which include virtuous habits, behaviors and observances (the "dos"). These virtues and ethical premises are considered in Hinduism as necessary for an individual to achieve a self-realized, enlightened, liberated state of existence (moksha).

Five Niyamas

In Patanjali's Yoga Sutras, the Niyamas are the second limb of the eight limbs of Yoga. Sadhana Pada Verse 32 lists the niyamas as:

1. Śauca: purity, clearness of mind, speech and body.
2. Santoṣa: contentment, acceptance of others and of one's circumstances as they are, optimism for self.
3. Tapas: austerity, self-discipline, persistent meditation, perseverance.
4. Svādhyāya: study of self, self-reflection, introspection of self's thoughts, speeches and actions.
5. Īśvarapraṇidhāna: contemplation of the Ishvara (God/Supreme Being, Brahman, True Self, Unchanging Reality), attunement to the supreme consciousness.

Ten Niyamas

In the diverse traditions and historical debate within Hinduism, some texts suggest a different and expanded list of *niyamas*. For example, the Shandilya and Varuha Upanishads, the Hatha Yoga Pradipika, verses 552 to 557 in Book 3 of the Tirumandhiram of Tirumular suggest ten *niyamas*, in the sense of positive duties, desirable behaviors and discipline. The Hatha Yoga Pradipika lists the ten niyamas in the following order, in verse 1.18,

1. Tapas: persistence, perseverance in one's purpose, austerity.
2. Santoṣa: contentment, acceptance of others and of one's circumstances as they are, optimism for self.
3. Āstika: faith in Real Self (jnana yoga, raja yoga), belief in God (bhakti yoga), conviction in Vedas/Upanishads (orthodox school).
4. Dāna: generosity, charity, sharing with others.
5. Īśvarapūjana: worship of the Ishvara (God/Supreme Being, Brahman, True Self, Unchanging Reality).
6. Siddhānta vakya śrāvaṇa: listening to the ancient scriptures.
7. Hrī: remorse and acceptance of one's past, modesty, humility.

8. Mati: think and reflect to understand, reconcile conflicting ideas.
9. Japa: mantra repetition, reciting prayers or knowledge.
10. Huta: rituals, ceremonies such as yajna sacrifice.

Some texts replace the last niyama of *Huta* with *Vrata*. The niyama of *Vrata* means making and keeping one's vows (resolutions), which may be pious observances. For example, a promise to fast and visit a pilgrimage site is a form of *Vrata*. The education process in ancient India, where Vedas and Upanishads were memorized and transmitted across generations without ever being written down, required a series of *Vrata* niyamas over a number of years.

Other Numbers of Niyamas

At least sixty five (65) ancient and medieval era Indian texts are known so far that discuss *Niyamas* and *Yamas*. Most are in Sanskrit, but some are in regional Indian languages of Hindus. The number of *Niyamas* mentioned in these texts range from just one to eleven, however 5 and 10 are the most common. The order of listed niyamas, the names and nature of each niyama, as well as the relative emphasis vary between the texts. For example, Sriprashna Samhita discusses only one Niyama in verse 3.22, and that Niyama being *Ahimsa*. Shivayoga Dipika, Sharada Tilaka, Vasishtha Samhita, Yoga Kalpalatika, Yajnavalkya Smriti and many others, each discuss ten *Niyamas*. Bhagavata Purana discusses eleven *Niyamas*, with kind hospitality of guests, to one's best ability, as an additional virtuous behavior. Other texts substitute one or more different concepts in their list of *Niyamas*. For example, in the five *Niyamas* listed by Markandeya Purana in verse 36.17, Matanga Parameshvaram in verse 17.31 and Pashupata Sutra in verse 1.9, each suggest Akrodha (non-anger) as a *Niyama*.

Many of the texts match Patanjali's five *Niyamas*. Ahimsa is the most widely discussed ethical theory, and highlighted as the highest virtue by majority of these texts.

Overlap Between Yamas and Niyamas

Some yamas (restraints, the "don'ts") are understood as reverse of niyamas (attitudes, behaviors, the "dos") in Hatha Yoga Pradipika. For example, *Ahimsa* and *Mitahara* are called as yama as well as niyama in verse 1.17 and 1.40. The text calls *Ahimsa* (nonviolence and non-injuring anyone by one's actions, words or in thoughts) as the highest virtuous habit, *Mitahara* (moderation in one's eating and drinking habits) as the best personal restraint, and Siddhasana as the foremost of Asanas in verse 1.40.

Buddhism

In Buddhist commentary (from the 5th to 13th centuries CE) we find the *pañcavidha niyama*, fivefold niyama which occurs in the following texts:

- In the *Aṭṭhasālinī* (272-274), the commentary attributed to Buddhaghosa on the *Dhammasangaṅi*, the first book of the Theravāda Abhidhamma Piṭaka.
- In the *Sumaṅgala-Vilāsinī* (DA 2.431), Buddhaghosa's commentary on the *Dīgha Nikāya*.
- In the *Abhidhammāvatāra* (PTS p.54), a verse summary of *Abhidhamma* by Buddhaghosa's contemporary, Buddhadatta.

- *Abhidhammamātika Internal Commentary*. (p. 58) The *Abhidhamma-mātika* is a matrix of abstracts for the Abhidhamma, with lists of pairs and triplets of terms from which the whole of the text can theoretically be reconstructed. The passage on the *niyamas* is from an internal commentary on the mātika associated with the Dhammasaṅgaṇī (the niyāmas don't appear to be mentioned in the mātrix itself, but only in this appendix.); and was composed in South India by Coḷaraṭṭha Kassapa (12th–13th century).
- *Abhidhammāvatāra-purāṇatīkā* (p.1.68). Composed by in Sri Lanka by Vācissara Mahāsāmi c. 13th century or Sāriputta c. 12th century. This text is a commentary on the text of the Abhidhammāvatāra Nāmarūpa-parichedo (ṭīka) so is technically a sub-sub-commentary. This commentary is an incomplete word by word commentary.

1. *utu-niyāma* "the constraint of the seasons", i.e. in certain regions of the earth at certain periods the flowering and fruiting of trees all at one time (*ekappahāreneva*), the blowing or ceasing of wind, the degree of the heat of the sun, the amount of rain-fall, some flowers like the lotuses opening during the day and closing at night and so on.
2. *bīja-niyāma* "the constraint of seeds or germs", i.e. a seed producing its own kind as barley seed produces barley.
3. *kammaniyāma* "the constraint of *kamma*", i.e. good actions produce good results and bad actions produce bad results. This constraint is said to be epitomised by [Dhammapada] verse 127 which explains that the consequences of actions are inescapable.
4. *citta-niyāma* "the constraint of mind", i.e. the order of the process of mind-activities as the preceding thought-moment causing and conditioning the succeeding one in a cause and effect relation.
5. *dhamma-niyāma* "the constraint of dhammas", i.e. such events like the quaking of the ten thousand world-systems at the Bodhisatta's conception in his mother's womb and at his birth. At the end of the discussion *Sumaṅgalavilāsinī* passage the Commentary says that *dhammaniyāma* explains the term dhammatā in the text of the *Mahāpadāna Sutta* (D ii.12) (Cf. S 12.20 for a discussion of the use of the word *dhammaniyamatā* in the suttas).

In these texts the fivefold *niyama* was introduced into commentarial discussions not to illustrate that the universe was intrinsically ethical but as a list that demonstrated the universal scope of *paṭicca-samuppāda*. The original purpose of expounding fivefold *niyama* was, according to Ledi Sayadaw, neither to promote or to demote the law of karma, but to show the scope of natural law as an alternative to the claims of theism.

C.A.F. Rhys Davids was the first western scholar to draw attention to the list of *pañcavidha niyama*, in her little book of 1912 entitled simply *Buddhism*. Her reason for mentioning it was to emphasise how for Buddhism we exist in a "moral universe" in which actions lead to just consequences according to a natural moral order, a situation she calls a "cosmodicy" in contrast with the Christian theodicy.

In Mrs Rhys Davids scheme the niyamas become:

- *kamma niyama*: ("action") consequences of one's actions.

- *utu niyama*: ("time, season") seasonal changes and climate, law of non-living matter.
- *bīja niyama*: ("seed") laws of heredity.
- *citta niyama*: ("mind") will of mind.
- *dhamma niyama*: ("law") nature's tendency to perfect.

This is similar to the scheme proposed by Ledi Sayadaw. Western Buddhist Sangharakshita has taken up Mrs Rhys Davids conception of the niyamas and made it an important aspect of his own teachings on Buddhism.

Spelling

In Pāli the word is spelled both *niyama* and *niyāma*, and the Pali Text Society Dictionary says that the two forms have become confused. It is likely that *niyāma* is from a causative form of the verb *ni√i*.

Ishvarapranidhana

Īśvarapraṇidhāna "commitment to the Īśvara ("Lord")" is also one of five Niyama (ethical observances) in Hinduism and Yoga.

Etymology and Meaning

Īśvarapraṇidhāna is a Sanskrit compound word composed of two words *īśvara* (**ईश्वर**) and *praṇidhāna* (**प्रणिधान**). *Īśvara* (sometimes spelled Īshvara) literally means "owner of best, beautiful", "ruler of choices, blessings, boons", or "chief of suitor, lover". Later religious literature in Sanskrit broadens the reference of this term to refer to God, the Absolute Brahman, True Self, or Unchanging Reality. *Praṇidhāna* is used to mean a range of senses including, "laying on, fixing, applying, attention (paid to), meditation, desire, prayer." In a religious translation of Patanjali's Eight-Limbed Yoga, the word *Īśvarapraṇidhāna* means committing what one does to a Lord, who is elsewhere in the Yoga Sūtras defined as a special person (puruṣa) who is the first teacher (paramaguru) and is free of all hindrances and karma. In more secular terms, it means acceptance, teachability, relaxing expectations, adventurousness.

Discussion

Yoga Sūtras of Patañjali

Īśvarapraṇidhāna is mentioned in the Yoga Sūtras of Patañjali as follows:

Sanskrit: **शौच संतोष तपः स्वाध्यायेश्वरप्रणिधानानि नियमाः ॥३२॥**

– Yoga Sutras II.32

This transliterates as, "Śauca, Santoṣa, Tapas, Svādhyāya and Īśvarapraṇidhāna are the Niyamas". This is the second limb in Patañjali's eight limb Yoga philosophy is called *niyamas* which include virtuous habits, behaviors and ethical observances (the "dos"). The Yoga Sutras of Patañjali use the term *Īśvara* in 11 verses: I.23 through I.29, II.1, II.2, II.32 and II.45. Patañjali defines *Īśvara* (Sanskrit: **ईश्वर**) in verse 24 of Book 1, as "a special Self (**पुरुषविशेष**, *puruṣa-viśeṣa*)",

Sanskrit: **क्लेश कर्म विपाकाशयैःपरामृष्टः पुरुषविशेष ईश्वरः ॥२४॥**

– Yoga Sutras I.24

This sutra of Yoga philosophy adds the characteristics of *Īśvara* as that special Self which is unaffected (**अपरामृष्ट**, *aparamrsta*) by one's obstacles/hardships (**क्लेश**, *klesha*), one's circumstances created by past or one's current actions (**कर्म**, *karma*), one's life fruits (**विपाक**, *vipâka*), and one's psychological dispositions/intentions (**आशय**, ashaya).

Īśvarapraṇidhāna is listed as the fifth niyama by Patañjali. In other forms of yoga, it is the tenth niyama. In Hinduism, the Niyamas are the "do list" and the Yamas are the "don't do" list, both part of an ethical theory for life.

Īśvara as a Metaphysical Concept

Hindu scholars have debated and commented on who or what is *Īśvara*. These commentaries range from defining Īśhvara from a "personal god" to "special self" to "anything that has spiritual significance to the individual". Ian Whicher explains that while Patañjali's terse verses can be interpreted both as theistic or non-theistic, Patañjali's concept of Īśvara in Yoga philosophy functions as a "transformative catalyst or guide for aiding the yogin on the path to spiritual emancipation". Desmarais states that Īśvara is a metaphysical concept in Yogasutras. *Īśvarapraṇidhāna* is investing, occupying the mind with this metaphysical concept. Yogasutra does not mention deity anywhere, nor does it mention any devotional practices (*Bhakti*), nor does it give Īśvara characteristics typically associated with a deity. In yoga sutras it is a logical construct, states Desmarais.

In verses I.27 and I.28, yogasutras associate Īśvara with the concept *Pranava* (**प्रणव, ॐ**) and recommends that it be repeated and contemplated in one of the limbs of eight step yoga. This is seen as a means to begin the process of dissociating from external world, connecting with one's inner world, focusing and getting one-minded in Yoga.

Whicher states that Patañjali's concept of Īśvara is neither a creator God nor the universal Absolute of Advaita Vedanta school of Hinduism. Whicher also notes that some theistic sub-schools of Vedanta philosophy of Hinduism, inspired by the Yoga school, prefer to explain the term *Īśvara* as the "Supreme Being that rules over the cosmos and the individuated beings". However, in the Yoga Sūtras of Patañjali, and extensive literature of Yoga school of Hinduism, Īśvara is not a Supreme Ruler, Īśvara is not an ontological concept, rather it has been an abstract concept to meet the pedagogical needs for human beings accepting Yoga philosophy as a way of life.

Īśvara as a Deity

Īśvarapraṇidhāna has been interpreted to mean the contemplation of a deity in some sub-schools of Hinduism. Zimmer in his 1951 Indian philosophies book noted that the Bhakti sub-schools, and its texts such as the Bhagavad Gita, refer to Isvara as a Divine Lord, or the deity of specific

Bhakti sub-school. Modern sectarian movements have emphasized Ishvara as Supreme Lord; for example, Hare Krishna movement considers Krishna as the Lord, Arya Samaj and Brahmoism movements – influenced by Christian and Islamic movements in India – conceptualize Ishvara as a monotheistic all powerful Lord. In traditional theistic sub-schools of Hinduism, such as the Vishishtadvaita Vedanta of Ramanuja and Dvaita Vedanta of Madhva, Ishvara is identified as Lord Vishnu/Narayana, that is distinct from the *Prakriti* (material world) and *Purusa* (soul, spirit). In all these sub-schools, *Īśvarapraṇidhāna* is the contemplation of the respective deity.

Radhakrishnan and Moore state that these variations in Īśvara concept is consistent with Hinduism's notion of "personal God" where the "ideals or manifestation of individual's highest Self values that are esteemed". *Īśvarapraṇidhāna*, or contemplation of Īśvara as a deity is useful, suggests Zaehner, because it helps the individual become more like Īśhvara. Riepe, and others, state that the literature of Yoga school of Hinduism neither explicitly defines nor implicitly implies, any creator-god; rather, it leaves the individual with freedom and choice of conceptualizing Īśvara in any meaningful manner he or she wishes, either in the form of "deity of one's choice" or "formless Brahman (Absolute Reality, Universal Principle, true special Self)". The need and purpose of Īśvara, whatever be the abstraction of it as "special kind of Self" or "personal deity", is not an end in itself, rather it is a means to "perfect the practice of concentration" in one's journey through the eight limbs of Yoga philosophy.

Īśvara as Pure Consciousness

Larson suggests Īśvara in *Īśvarapraṇidhāna* can be understood through its chronological roots. Yoga school of Hinduism developed on the foundation of Samkhya school of Hinduism. In the non-theistic/atheistic Samkhya school, *Purusa* is a central metaphysical concept, and envisioned as "pure consciousness". Further, *Purusa* is described by Samkhya school to exist in a "plurality of pure consciousness" in its epistemological theory (rather than to meet the needs of its ontological theory). In the Yoga Sutras, Patanjali defines *Īśhvara* as a "special Purusa" in verse I.24, with certain characteristics. Īśhvara, then may be understood as one among the plurality of "pure consciousness", with characteristics as defined by Patanjali in verse I.24.

Īśvara as Spiritual but not Religious

Van Ness, and others, suggests that the concepts of Īśvara, Īśvara-pranidhana and other limbs of Yoga may be pragmatically understood as "spiritual but not religious".

Pratyahara

Pratyahara (Devanāgarī प्रत्याहार, Tibetan སོ་སོར་སྡུད་པ་, Wylie *so sor sdud pa*) or the 'withdrawal of the senses' is the fifth element among the Eight stages of Patanjali's Ashtanga Yoga, as mentioned in his classical work, *Yoga Sutras of Patanjali* composed in the 2nd century BCE. It is also the first stage of the six-branch yoga (*ṣaḍaṅgayoga*) of the Buddhist Kālacakra tantra, where it refers to the withdrawal of the five senses from external objects to be replaced by the mentally created senses of an enlightened deity. This phase is roughly analogous to the physical isolation (*kāyaviveka*, Tib. *lus bden*) phase of Guhyasamāja tantra.

For Patanjali, it is a bridge between the *bahiranga* (external) aspects of yoga namely, yama, niyama, asana, pranayama, and the *antaranga* (internal) yoga. Having actualized the *pratyahara* stage, a practitioner is able to effectively engage into the practice of Samyama. At the stage of *pratyahara*, the consciousness of the individual is internalized in order that the sensations from the senses of taste, touch, sight, hearing and smell don't reach their respective centers in the brain and takes the *sadhaka* (practitioner) to next stages of Yoga, namely Dharana (concentration) and Dhyana (meditation), and Samadhi (mystical absorption), being the aim of all Yogic practices.

Etymology

Pratyahara is derived from two Sanskrit words: *prati* and *ahara*, with ahara meaning food, or anything taken into ourselves, and prati, a preposition meaning away or against. Together they mean "weaning away from ahara", or simply ingestion

Types of Pratyahara

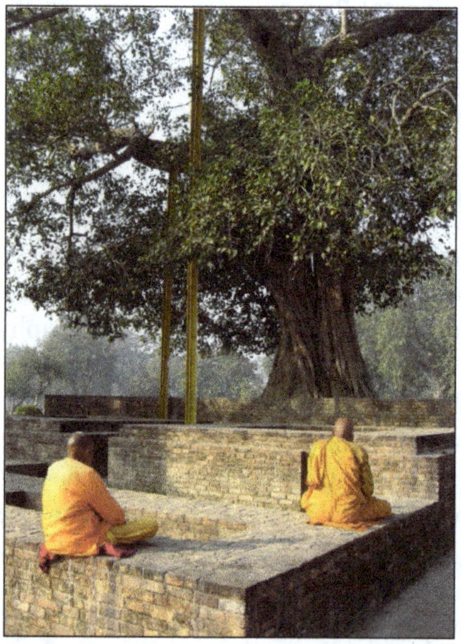

Monks meditating under the Anandabodhi tree in *Jetavana Monastery*, Sravasti.

Withdrawal of Senses or Indriya Pratyahara

This involves withdrawal of senses, or sensory inputs into our physical being, coming from our five senses, namely organs creating a sensory overload, and hence hinders collection of the mind, as in Dharana, the next stage of Yoga.

Withdrawal of Prana or Prana Pratyahara

Control of our senses requires mastery over the flow of prana, as that is what drives the senses. To stop the scattering of valuable vital energy of the body or prana, we need to seek control over its flow, and harmonize it. This is done through various practices including bringing the entire focus to a single point in the body.

These two lead to the subsequent two types of pratyahara, the Control of Action or 'Karma pratyahara', which entails not just control of motor organs, but also right action or work, and Karma Yoga, surrender of every action to the divine and performing it as an act of service. This leads to the final form of pratyahara - the Withdrawal of Mind or 'Mano pratyahara', which is practiced by consciously withdrawing attention from anything that is unwholesome, and distracting for the mind such as by withdrawing attention from the senses, and directing it inwards.

Practices in Pratyahara

One of the most common practices for Pratyahara is Pranayama, wherein we automatically withdraw from the external and bring our focus inwards towards our breath, as connection with the external senses and stimuli are all severed gradually.

Apart from Pranayama, another method that is used to aid in the development of Pratyahara is to concentrate on the point between the eyebrows. This location is known as Ajna Chakra or the third eye.

Another common technique for inducing Pratyahara is to first reduce physical stimuli, then concentrate on one sense, such as hearing. The mind has a natural tendency to roam between the sensory inputs. In this situation, as there are no longer any other significant sensory inputs, when the mind gets tired of hearing, it is forced to turn inward.

At the advanced levels, the currents which pulsate through the nerves and even the involuntary muscles are turned off by the practitioner. This may also be accomplished through Pranayama or breath-control.

References

- Ray, Reginald A. (2002). Indestructibe Truth: The Living Spirituality of Tibetan Buddhism - The World of Tibetan Buddhism Volume One. Boston, Massachusetts, U.S.A.: Shambala Publications, Inc. ISBN 1-57062-910-2. P.124
- "Religion in Spain". Sahaja Worldwide News and Announcements (SWAN). sahajayoga.org. Vishwa Nirmala Dharma. 19 July 2006. Retrieved 26, June 2020
- "Experience Your Self Realization". sahajayoga.org. Vishwa Nirmala Dharma. 12 June 2006. Archived from the original on 19 November 2011. Retrieved 26, May 2020
- Sturgess, Stephen (2014). Yoga editation: Still Your Mind and Awaken Your Inner Spirit. Oxford, UK: Watkins Publishing Limited. pp. 18–19. ISBN 978-1-78028-644-0
- "Historic video affirming the role of World Council for the Advancement of Sahaja Yoga". Sahaja Worldwide Announcements and News (SWAN). sahajayoga.org. Vishwa Nirmala Dharma. Retrieved 26, August 2020
- "Shri Mataji Radiates A Divine Energy". sahajayoga.org. Vishwa Nirmala Dharma. Archived from the original on 3 December 2011. Retrieved 11, June 2020
- "List of ECOSOC/Beijing and New Accredited NGOs that attended the special session of the General Assembly". un.org. United Nations. Retrieved 20, January 2020
- Ray, Nihar Ranjan (October 2000). "The concept of 'Sahaj' in Guru Nanak's theology". The Sikh Review. 48 (562). Archived from the original on 27 September 2011. Retrieved 26,June 2020
- Subramuniya (2003). Merging with Śiva: Hinduism's contemporary metaphysics. Himalayan Academy Publications. p. 155. ISBN 9780945497998. Retrieved 06, April 2020

- Mallinson, James (2004). The Gheranda samhita: the original Sanskrit and an English translation. YogaVidya.com. p. 16. ISBN 978-0-9716466-3-6. Retrieved 10, April 2020
- Barba, Eugenio; Savarese, Nicola (1991). A dictionary of theatre anthropology: the secret art of the performer. London, United Kingdom: Routledge. p. 136. ISBN 0-415-05308-0
- "Teachers and Aunties Needed for International Sahaja School at Canajoharie". Sahaja Worldwide Announcements and News (SWAN). sahajayoga.org. Vishwa Nirmala Dharma. 2 December 2006. Retrieved 20, May 2020
- Patanjali (2003). The Yoga-Sutra of Patanjali: A New Translation with Commentary. Shambhala Classics. Translated by Chip Hartranft. ISBN 1-59030-023-8
- Tatke, Vinita (February 2000). "Case Study Civil Society & Governance Project". Archived from the original on 2004-01-03. Retrieved 06, July 2020
- Michael Palmer and Stanley Burgess (2012), The Wiley-Blackwell Companion to Religion and Social Justice, John Wiley & Sons, ISBN 978-1405195478
- "Message to all the Sahaja Yogis of the world from Arneau, Coordinator of the World Council". sahajayoga.org.in. Archived from the original on 29 September 2011. Retrieved 11, August 2020
- "The Opening of Canajoharie Sahaja School". Sahaja Worldwide Announcements and News (SWAN). sahajayoga.org. Vishwa Nirmala Dharma. 28 July 2004. Retrieved 26, August 2020
- "A Wonderful Evening with Shri Mataji". Sahaja Worldwide Announcements and News (SWAN). sahajayoga.org. Vishwa Nirmala Dharma. 10 July 2005. Retrieved 19, April 2020
- Verse 46, chapter II; for translation referred: "Patanjali Yoga Sutras" by Swami Prabhavananda , published by the Sri Ramakrishna Math ISBN 81-7120-221-7 p. 111

5

Pranayama and its Types

The practice within yoga which focuses on breathing is known as pranayama. It involves complete suspension of breathing. Some of the major forms of pranayama are bhastrika pranayama, anuloma pranayama, bahya pranayama and bhramari pranayama. This chapter discusses in detail these forms of pranayama.

Pranayama is the perfect control of the life-currents through control of breath, and is the process by which we understand the secret of prana and manipulate it. You can hardly make any spiritual progress without the practice of pranayama. One who has grasped this prana has grasped the very core of cosmic life and activity. Through various exercises and training in pranayama the yogi tries to realize in this little body the whole of cosmic life, and attain perfection.

Breath is a physical aspect or external manifestation of prana, the vital force, and thus pranayama begins with the regulation of the breath. Breath, like electricity, is gross prana, while prana itself is subtle. By controlling the breath you can control the prana– just as you can control the other wheels by controlling or stopping the fly wheel of a diesel engine, and just as you can control the hairspring, cog wheels and the main spring of a watch by controlling the minute hand. Control of breath is achieved through manipulation of the lungs and the breathing process.

The Lungs and the Breathing Process

The organs of respiration consist of two lungs, one on either side of the chest and the air passages that lead to them. The lungs are located in the upper thoracic cavity of the chest, one on each side of the median line, and are separated from each other by the heart, the greater blood vessels and the larger air tubes. The lungs are spongy, porous, and their tissues are very elastic, containing innumerable air-sacs or alveoli. Each lung consists of an apex and a base. The base is directed towards the diaphragm, the muscular septum, the dividing wall between chest and the abdomen.

The air passage consists of the interior of the nose, pharynx or throat, larynx or voice box, trachea or windpipe, right and left bronchi and the smaller bronchial tubes. When we breathe, we draw in the air through the nose and after it has passed through the pharynx and larynx, it passes into the windpipe, thence into the right and left bronchial tubes, which in turn, subdivide into innumerable smaller tubes called bronchioles, which terminate in minute subdivisions in the millions of small air-sacs of the lungs. When spread out over an unbroken surface, these air-sacs of the lungs would cover an area of 1,40,000 square feet.

The air is drawn into the lungs by the action of the diaphragm. When it expands, the size of the chest and the lungs is increased and the outside air rushes into the vacuum thus created. The chest and lungs contract when the diaphragm relaxes and the air is expelled from the lungs.

The lungs purify the blood. The blood starts in its arterial journey, bright red and richly laden with life-giving qualities and properties. It returns by the venous route, blue, laden with the waste matter of the system. From the right side of the heart the impure blood goes to the lungs, for purification. It is distributed among the millions of tiny air cells of the lungs. A breath of air is inhaled and the oxygen of the air comes in contact with the impure blood through the thin walls of the hair-like blood vessels of the lungs called pulmonary capillaries. The walls of the capillaries are very thin, like muslin cloth, and thus oxygen easily penetrates through the walls of these thin capillaries.

When the oxygen comes in contact with the tissues, a form of combustion takes place. The blood takes up oxygen and releases carbonic acid gas generated from the waste products and poisonous matter which have been gathered by the blood from all parts of the system. The purified blood passes into the different arteries of the body. It is estimated that in a day 35,000 pints of blood traverse the capillaries of the lungs for purification.

By controlling the motion of the lungs or respiratory organs, we can control the prana that is vibrating inside. The mind is fastened to prana, like a bird to a string; therefore, by control of prana, the mind can be easily controlled. Just as the bird that is tied to a post by a string, after flying here and there, finds its resting place on the post, so also this mind-bird after running hither and thither, to various sensual objects, finds its resting place during deep sleep in prana.

Pranayama

The following timeline gives a general bird's eye overview of the history of pranayama practices. Though this list is neither intended to be exhaustive nor comprehensive in its scope, it includes a small number of key texts that will be of interest to anyone who wishes to learn more about the history and practice of pranayama.

Brihadaranyaka Upanishad

While references to the the term prana can be found as early as 3,000 BCE in the Chandogya Upanishad, references to pranayama as a breathing practice do not occur until much later in yogic literature (approximately 700 BCE).

One of the earliest recorded references to pranayama as a breath related practice can be found in hymn 1.5.23 of the Brihadaranyaka Upanishad. Clearly linking breathing practices to the regulation of vital energy and life-force, the Upanishad states:

"One should indeed breathe in (arise), but one should also breathe out (without setting) while saying, "Let not the misery that is dying reach me." When one would practice that (breathing), one should rather desire to thoroughly realize that (immortality). It is rather through that (realization) that he wins a union with this divinity (breath), that is a sharing of worlds."

No additional guidelines for pranayama practice are given in this Upanishad. However, the idea that breathing could be used to achieve greater health and even immortality is a theme that is often repeated in subsequent yogic texts and teachings.

The Bhagavad Gita

References to pranayama practices can also be found in the Bhagavad Gita, Chapter 4, verse 29. The text highlights the use of conscious inhaling, exhaling and breath retention to effect trancelike states. The text also suggests that the regular practice of pranayama can be used to enact greater control over the senses by "curtailing the eating process."

The Maitrayaniya Upanishad

The Maitrayaniya Upanishad is an important text in the history of pranayama because it contains one of the earliest references to pranayama as a component in a larger, multifaceted system. Most likely composed centuries before the Yoga Sutras of Patanjali, this text enumerates yoga as a six-step process of breath control (pranayama), sensory withdrawal (pratyahara), concentration (dharana), meditation (dhyana), reasoning (tarka) and union (samadhi).

Specific references to pranayama practices can be found in chapter six, verse 21. The text states that deliverance can be accomplished by using a combination of breath retention practices and concentration on the sacred syllable Om in order to redirect prana into the body's central energy channel (Sushumna).

Circa 100 to 400 CE

Most scholars agree that the Yoga Sutras of Patanjali are a compilation of texts from earlier yoga traditions. By the time of Patanjali, yoga as a system had continued to adapt and grow. The six-limbed system mentioned in the Maitrayaniya Upanishad had grown into eight limbed approach that included asana (physical postures) yama and niyama (social and ethical precepts) pranayama as well as four additional stages of meditative absorption (pratyahara, dharana, dhyana and samadhi).

References to pranayama can be found in verses 2.29 – thru 2.53 of the Sutras. While Patanjali does not go deeply into the nature of prana in these sections, he does detail four separate aspects of the breath: inhale, exhale and retention. In addition, Patanajali also makes reference to a fourth pranayama in sutra 2.51 that he claims surpasses or goes beyond the other three.

In addition, Patanjali notes a number of specific benefits of pranayama practice. These benefits include mental fitness and the ability to concentrate – a prerequisite to deeper states of yoga practice. Additionally, Patanjali states in verse 2:52 that regular pranayama practice could lessen or dissolve the veil that covers our "inner illumination."

The Hatha Yoga Pradipika

Though traditionalists trace the roots of Hatha Yoga practice to the God Shiva, many scholars associate the founding of the Hatha yoga movement with the Maha Siddha Goraksha Nath. Widely associated with being the founding father of the practice, Gorakshanath is purported to have lived sometime between the 10th and 15th century CE. Numerous texts are accredited to him and his disciples.

One of the most important texts of the medieval era is the Hatha Yoga Pradipika, which was written by Goraksha Nath's pupil Swami Svatmarama. Drawing from earlier systems, the text emphasizes the attainment of good heath and spiritual realization through a combination of physical postures, pranayama practices and meditative contemplations.

The Pradipika differs from some of the early texts in the history of pranayama, because it more fully details actual instructions for practice. These instructions include specific references to alternate nostril-breathing patterns, details on how to retain the breath, guidelines on auspicious times for practice and an overview of the various signs of progress in pranayama.

Further references to pranayama techniques can be found in a number of additional medieval manuscripts. The most important of these texts include the Gheranda Samhita (late seventeenth century) and Shiva Samhita (seventeenth or eighteenth century CE).

Pranayama Today

While most modern pranayama practices are based at least in part on their original counterparts, contemporary pranayama practices often include a number of additional variations on the basic breathing patterns found in the earlier texts mentioned in this paper.

Modern variants on the practice tend to integrate a combination of modern anatomical knowledge with more traditional yogic teachings in order to refine technique and better explain the physiological and psychological processes that occur when practicing pranayama.

The most notable example of this new approach to pranayama practices can be found in the book "Light on Pranayama", by the the late B.K.S. Iyengar. A seminal text on modern day pranayama practice, Iyengar's book is a must read for any student with an interest in the history of pranayama.

The Importance of Pranayama in Yoga Practice

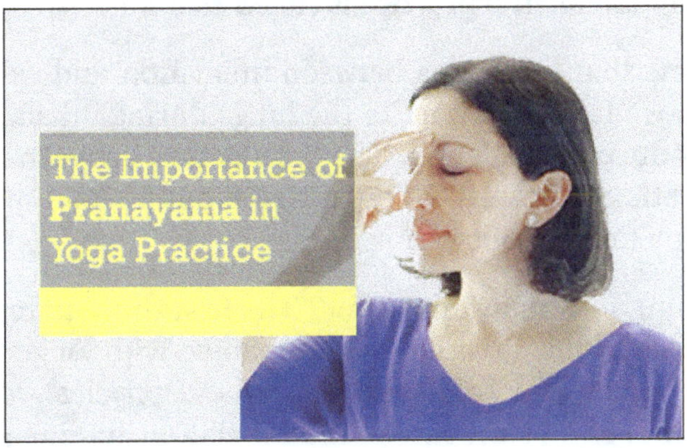

Pranayama is a significant part of yoga and involves specific breathing techniques and exercises. The word Pranayama has been derived from two Sanskrit words, "Prana" and "Ayama", where "Prana" means "life force" or "life energy" and "Ayama" means "control of". So then, the term Pranayama communicates to us control and expansion of prana. Pranayama is the fourth of the eight limbs of yoga, the structural framework of yoga practice as laid down by Patanjali, in his Yoga Sutras.

"Prana" is spoken of, as the culmination of all energy manifested in the universe. Basically, the force or energy which sustains life. It also encompasses the hidden forces that govern various universal phenomenon like light, heat, magnetism etc.

The prana within us is expressed by our breath, that is outside of us. We can regulate the prana within by taking control of our breath. The atmosphere and the cosmos all about us are abundantly full of prana. When we learn to breathe deeply, correctly and mindfully we ingest more vast doses of this dynamic energy. Slowing and controlling the breath helps steady the mind. A troubled or overactive mind can be brought to a state of calmness. Mastering the mind enables us to strengthen our will.

So, when we speak of Pranayama, it does not merely involve breathing techniques and exercises. It is, in fact, the art and science of mind ful living. The breath is the core of what we think, how we act and what we truly are. It is the window to the deepest layers of our mind. Pranayama helps us to access the depth of our mind and expand our horizons to harmonize with the ever-expanding universe.

The basic philosophy of the practice of Pranayama is that the flow of life in and out of us is governed by the breath. So, regulating the breath through Pranayama molds our inner being keeping us in a state of balance.

Composition of Pranayama

Pranayama encompasses working consciously with the breath. It has three components to it namely controlled inhalation, (in Sanskrit 'Puraka')controlled exhalation (in Sanskrit 'Rechaka') and holding of the breath, (in Sanskrit 'Kumbhaka') The process of putting all three components into practice is called "Sahita".

Breathing is a process that alternates between inhalation and exhalation. This takes place in cycles when we take in oxygen to the lungs during inhalation and release out stale noxious gasses during exhalation. The brief gap in between that lasts a few seconds is where respiration takes place. We respire about fifteen times a minute and the instance of respiration takes about four seconds.

So, how does breathing in Pranayama differ? The first thing to remember is exhaling heavy and inhaling light. Slow breathing accompanied with longer exhalation ensures better control over breath and enhances mental and physical relaxation. Have you heard your yoga teacher say, "Take care of the exhalation and inhalation will take care of itself"? It is a common perception that inhalation is more important, but that is not the case.

Pranayama stresses upon "letting go" during an exhale. When you are breathing out, you are releasing and letting go. It takes the least effort. While exhaling long and heavy, give yourself completely to your breath and relax just like you do at the end of a hard day's work.

When you inhale deeply, you lighten up your mind. Pranayama utilizes this set of simple ideas. These contending forces of inhalation and exhalation work together to bring out the compound effect in Pranayama.

The second aspect in Pranayama is awareness or mindfulness When we take deep long breaths, we are aware of breathing in and breathing out. We focus Just on the breathing, which keeps us rooted in the present moment and we begin to realize –this moment is all encompassing. This present moment is all we have and is most important. We have kept away from worrying or fretting over past and future. We feel relaxed and light which enhances circulation of blood and oxygen.

Inhalation, Exhalation and Retention

Pranayama has three components: the external breath, the internal breath and the steady state in between the two. When the breath is expired, it is rechaka, the first kind of pranayama. When the breath is drawn in, it is the second, termed pooraka. When the breath is suspended, it is the third kind, called kumbhaka, or retention of breath.

Kumbhaka increases the life-span of an individual. It augments the inner spiritual force, vigour and vitality. If you retain the breath for one minute, this one minute is added to your span of life. By taking the breath to the brahmarandhra, the fontanelle at the top of the head (said to be the connecting point between the spirit and the body) and keeping it there, the yogi can defeat the lord of death, Yama, and conquer death.

In the practice of pranayama, rechaka, pooraka and kumbhaka, are controlled and regulated by space, time and number.

The Space of the Breath

'Space' refers to whether the breath is inside or outside of the body, the length of the breath, and if the prana is held in some particular part of the body. During both inhalation and exhalation, the distance to which the breath extends inside or outside the body varies. This variation accords with the tattwa which is pervading at the time of practice. The length of the breath is respectively 12, 16, 4, 8, 0 angulas, finger-breadths, according to whether the tattwa– prithvi, apas, tejas, vayu or akasha (earth, water, fire, air, ether or space) is predominant at that time.

The 'place' or 'space' of exhalation lies within 12 angulas of the tip of the nose. This can be measured using a piece of reed or cotton. The place of inhalation ranges from the head down to the soles of the feet and can be felt through a sensation similar to the touch of an ant. The place of kumbhaka consists of the places of both exhalation and inhalation combined, because the breath can be retained at either or both of these places.

The Time of Breath

The duration of the inhalation, exhalation or retention is generally counted in matras (approximately a second). But here the 'time' also refers to how long the prana should be fixed in a particular centre or part. There are three types of pranayama categorized by duration: adhama or inferior, madhyama middle and uttama superior. Vachaspati describes them thus, "Measured by 36 matras, is the first attempt, udghata, which is mild. Twice that is the second, which is middling. Thrice that is the third, which is intense. This is the pranayama as measured by number."

Adhama pranayama consists of a count of 12 matras, madhyama consists of 24 matras and the uttama occupies a time of 32 matras. This count is for pooraka in each case.

The ratio between pooraka, kumbhaka and rechaka is 1:4:2. So, if you inhale for a period of 12 matras you will have to maintain kumbhaka for a period of 48 matras and then the time for rechaka will be 24 matras. This count is for adhama pranayama, but the same rule applies to the other two varieties.

Extending the matra needs to be done gradually, first practise adhama for a month, then madhyama for three months, and finally begin uttama.

Number of Pranayama

'Number' refers to the number of times the pranayama is performed, and thus is long or short according to the period of time it is practised. Just as water, thrown on a hot pan shrivels upon all sides as it is being dried up, so also air, moving in or out ceases its action by a strong effort of restraint in kumbhaka, and stays within. The yogic student should slowly take the number of pranayamas up to 80 in one sitting. He should have four sittings: in the morning, noon, evening and midnight, and should practise thus 320 pranayamas in all.

Seat of Prana

The seat of Prana is heart. Though the Antahkarana is one, yet it assumes four forms, viz., (i) Manas, (ii) Buddhi, (iii) Chitta and (iv) Ahamkara according to the different functions it performs. Likewise, though Prana is one, it assumes five forms viz., (1) Prana, (2) Apana, (3) Samana, (4) Udana and (5) Vyana according to the different functions it performs. This is termed as Vritti Bheda. The principal Prana is called Mukhya Prana. The Prana, joined with Ahamkara, lives in the heart. Of these five, Prana and Apana are the chief agents.

The seat of Prana is the heart; of Apana, the anus; of Samana, the region of the naval; of Udana, the throat; while Vyana is all-pervading. It moves all over the body.

These are the four stages of Pranayama:

- Arambha: the commencement stage wherein the person's interest in Pranayama is awakened.
- Ghata: the stage where the three saris merge to envelope the soul. The three sariras are gross, subtle, and causal.
- Parichay: the stage where the yogi experiences the knowledge of Pranayama.
- Nispatti: the stage where the yogi goes beyond his physical body, and unites with the supreme.

Performing Pranayama Yoga

Pranayama techniques are best practiced while sitting on the floor on a folded blanket. This form of practice is applicable to padmasana also. However; any other posture will do provided the back is kept erect from the base of the spine to the neck and perpendicular to the floor. Bad and poorly performed posture will lead to shallow breathing and low endurance. One must empty the bladder and bowels before starting pranayama yoga.

Pranayama yoga must be performed in empty stomach. The best time for practice is the early morning, preferably before sunrise when the pollution is at its lowest level, and the body and brain are still free. However, if morning is unsuitable, pranayama may be practiced after sunset, when the air is cool and pleasant. The place suitable for all kinds of Yoga must be clean and calm.

Reduced Breathing Rate

With yoga breathing you can train yourself to breathe more slowly and more deeply. You can reduce your breathing rate from about fifteen breaths a minute to 5-6 breaths a minute, which amounts to reducing the breathing rate by one third. Reduced breathing rate leads to:

- Slowing down the heart rate as more oxygen can be pumped even with less number of breaths. Follow the ration of 1:2 for inhalation:exhalation.
- Reduced wear and tear of internal organs.
- Lowering of blood pressure, relaxation of body tensions and quieter nerves.

Pranayama Practice Increases Life

As per yoga philosophy, longevity depends on your breathing rate. Lowering of breathing rate is likely to increase your life. For example, a tortoise takes four to five breaths in a minute and it lives up to 200 years or more.

Blood Circulation Improves

As a result of breathing, the freshly oxygenated blood (during inhalation) travels from lungs to the heart. The heart pumps it via arteries and blood vessels to every part of the body, where in turn it seeps into every tissue and cell. This improves the blood circulation and more oxygen/prana or cosmic energy reaches all parts of your body.

Pranayama for Healthy Heart

Our heart is the most industrious organ of our body. The heart beats 100,000 times a day. It is pumping blood day in and day out non-stop all your life. The health of your heart determines your life expectancy and quality of life in old age. More oxygen in the blood means more oxygen to muscles of the heart.

Benefits of Pranayama for Functioning of Body Organs

- Better functioning of autonomic system improves the working of lungs, heart, diaphragm, abdomen, intestines, kidneys and pancreas.

- Digestive system improves and diseases pertaining to digestive organs are cured.
- General irritability due to lethargy/fatigue vanishes.
- By pranayama practice all body organs gets more oxygen, toxins are removed from body, therefore onset of various diseases is prevented. Pranayama strengthens the immune system.

Better Mental Health

Pranayama practice provides freedom from negative and harmful mental conditions like anger, depression, lasciviousness, greed for money, arrogance etc.

With pranayama fluctuations of mind are controlled and it prepares the mind for meditation. With practice of pranayama, you will start experiencing lightness of body, feeling of inner peace, better sleep, better memory and better concentration whereby improving the spiritual powers/skills.

Better Breathing Improves Quality of Life in Old Age

As a person with sedentary lifestyle reaches middle age, lung tissues tend to grow less and less elastic and lung capacity decreases. Pranayama can help to reduce the effects of following old age problems:

- Loss of vitality.
- Accumulation of uric acid in the blood stream which often leads to frequent joint pains and discomfort.
- Backaches, headaches, rheumatism, stiffening muscles and joints.
- Proper circulation of blood is impeded by a sluggish diaphragm or hardening arteries.

It is recommended to start learning pranayama from a yoga teacher without any delay in order to experience the immense benefits of pranayama. Benefits of yoga breathing can be realised only by experience. Establish a daily routine of yoga breathing exercises. If you want to start on your own, first start with rhythmic deep breathing to get into the rhythm.

Precautions for Pranayama Practice

1. If you have any chronic medical condition, seek advice of your doctor and yoga teacher before starting pranayama.
2. Pranayama should be practiced only after one has gained control over body by mastering the asanas. Pranayama practice generates prana energy in the body

and yoga asana practice removes the blockages of nadis which conducts prana energy throughout the body.

3. Always breathe through the nose unless specifically asked to do so.
4. There should not be any strain during pranayama practice. Lungs are delicate organ; ensure that your breathing is not forced beyond limits.
5. Do not make loud sounds during breathing. Keep the breath rhythmic and steady.
6. Pranayama should not be practiced immediately after meals. You can do pranayama at least three hours after meals. Remember a heavy meal will take much longer to get digested. For example if you do pranayama in evening, eat a healthy lunch which gets digested by the time you start pranayama.
7. Beginners should not hold breath. When you become comfortable with basics of pranayama, learn to hold breath under the guidance of an expert teacher after mastering the basics of yoga breathing.
8. If you feel tiredness or discomfort, stop doing pranayama, lie down in shavasana while carrying out normal breathing. Consult your yoga teacher before starting with pranayama again.
9. Do not practice pranayama if you are too tired, relax for 10-15 minutes in shavasana before doing pranayama.
10. If you do yoga asanas and pranayama, practice yoga asanas before pranayama. After practicing asanas, relax in shavasana before doing pranayama. Do not do any strenuous exercise after pranayama.
11. Pranayama should not be practiced in a hurry.
12. Do pranayama outdoors or in a well ventilated room.
13. Pranayama should not be practiced when the lungs are congested.

Kapalbhati, bhastrika pranayama is prohibited for people suffering from heart disease, high blood pressure or hernia. For kapalabhati, exhalation must be gentle for beginners, do not use excessive force.

Shitkari pranayama is prohibited for people with low blood pressure. Do not practice this pranayama in winters.

Do not do Suryabhedi in summers and Chandrabhedi in winters.

Agnisar Pranayama should not be done by people with hernia, high blood pressure and also not after any stomach surgery.

Bhastrika Pranayama

Bhastrika Pranayama is one of the main forms of Pranayama. In Sanskrit, Bhastrika means the 'bellows '. Just as the blacksmith blows his bellows to create heat and purify iron, Bhastrika is said to purify the mind and clear pranic blocks. Bhastrika is mentioned in the yoga texts Hatha Yoga Pradeepika and the Gheranda Samhita.

Bhastrika involves both rapid inhalation as well as exhalation. This helps to increase the circulation of blood in the entire body. During rapid and forced exhalation, the chest is compressed, thereby pushing the blood towards the head. During the inhalation, the reverse takes place. This process increases the blood flow to every part of the body, increasing the vitality of all the organs and tissues. Long term practice of Bhastrika purifies the body and awakens the inherent higher powers. During Bhastrika, the increase in blood flow causes a slight rise in body temperature, accompanied with mild sweating which reduces the temperature and keeps the body at normal temperature. Most pranayama techniques either increase or decrease the body temperature, but Bhastrika more or less maintains the body temperature. Bhastrika also increases the oxygen content in the blood.

Bhastrika practice can be considered as a combination of Kapalbhati and Ujjayi pranayama. The exhalation is similar to that in Kapalbhati and inhalation is similar to that done in Ujjayi pranayama. Once you have practiced Kapalbhati and Ujjayi, Bhastrika is easy. Bhastrika can be practiced both in the morning and evening. During summer, if the temperature is high, the practice should be restricted to mornings only. Bhastrika is an advanced practice and should be done on an empty stomach, after evacuation in the morning. Those who take up prolonged practice of Bhastrika, should take only light meals during morning and night. The lunch can be normal.

Limitations of Bhastrika Pranayama

Those suffering from heart diseases should not do this pranayama. Also avoid it when you have a severe block of the nose. Those with acute asthma and fever should also not attempt Bhastrika. If you had any recent surgery, please consult your doctor before attempting Bhastrika. Practice of Bhastrika can be little intense for some people. It should be learned only under the guidance of a qualified yoga instructor. In case of any existing medical conditions, please consult your doctor before taking up the practice.

Performing Bhastrika Pranayama

Sit in any steady asana. Padmasana, Siddhasana and Vajrasana are ideal for the practice.

1. Keep the body erect and close the mouth.

2. Inhale and exhale in rapid succession. During this process a hissing sound is produced. Start with say 10 inhalations and exhalations per round. It can be increased over a period of time. Some practitioners even do it till they get perspiration.

3. Some practice Bhastrika along with Kumbhaka (holding of the breath) at the end of the last exhalation. To do this, take a deep breath after the last exhalation and hold the breath inside for as long as comfortable. Then exhale and start breathing normally. This will constitute one round. Another way of doing it is mentioned in Hatha Yoga Pradeepika. There it is said that at the end of the last exhalation, one should breathe in through the right nostril and hold the breath. Then release the breath through the left nostril.

4. Do three such rounds of Bhastrika Between the rounds, rest for a while, till the breathing comes back to normal. If you are short of time, practice at least one round which is good enough to maintain fitness.

5. Have two sittings, one in the morning and one in the evening (if the temperature is cool).

Benefits of Bhastrika Pranayama

Bhastrika pranayama increases the oxygen content in the blood. Extra oxygen replenishes the entire body.

1. It removes blockages in the nose and chest.

2. It is good for asthma patients and removes inflammation of the throat.

3. Bhastrika increases the gastric fire and improves appetite.

4. Bhastrika when practiced with Kumbhaka can generate heat in the body and keep it warm in cold weather.

5. Bhastrika improves general health and activates all the organs.

6. Bhastrika purifies the nadis or the energy (pranic) channels in the body, ensuring free flow of prana to all the organs in the body.

7. Bhastrika has great spiritual benefits. It helps to break through the three Granthis or psychic knots that bind the soul. The three knots are called Brahma Granthi (at the base of spine, near Mooladhara and Swadhishtana Chakra), Vishnu Granthi (around the heart chakra) and Rudra Granthi (at the Agna Chakra). These are emotional and mental knots, block the individual's evolution. Prolonged practice of Bhastrika loosens up these Granthis. Bhastrika destroys the phlegm that blocks the entrance to Sushumna Nadi (or the central

pranic channel), thus enabling energy to pass up the spinal channel. Prolonged practice can help to awaken the inherent Kundalini Shakti at the base of the spine.

8. Bhastrika destroys the defects of Vata (wind), Pitta (Bile) and Kapha (Phlegm) and balances these three.

Bhastrika is one of the main practices taken up by serious students of yoga. One should not overdo the exercise out of enthusiasm. Start with less rounds (say 10 inhalations and exhalations). Slowly increase it to 60 or 120 over a period of time. Some do even 500 or more, depending on the strength and comfort of the practitioner. Some do it till they get tired and start to perspire. One should judge one's own capacity before doing it. Those who take up Bhastrika seriously should eat only Satvic food (pure, fresh, light, nourishing and easy to digest). also, the use of enema is recommended to keep the bowels clean, whenever required.

There are many variations of Bhastrika. In some variations, only one nostril is used for inhalation and exhalation. First it is done through the left nostril and then through the right nostril. In another variation, the inhalation is done through one nostril and the exhalation is done through the other.

Precautions to be Taken While Practicing Bhastrika Pranayama

- You might feel a little dizzy or pukish sensation after practicing Bhastrika pranayama because of excessive perspiration. So, it is advised to not make very loud sounds while inhaling during the practice.
- Facial contortions and excessive shaking of the body should be avoided while practicing Bhastrika pranayama. But after repeated practice, you experience that you cannot stop these signs, you must consult a trained yoga expert for guidance.
- Bhastrika pranayama consumes a lot of physical energy during the practice, so it is advised for the beginners to take small rest in between rounds while practicing. Also, it should be practiced slowly and people should not rush into doing it very fast or rushing into advanced practice as you can reap maximum benefits from the practice by doing it slowly.

Contra-Indications While Practicing Bhastrika Pranayama

- Bhastrika should not be practiced by people who suffer from high blood pressure.
- People with heart disease should also not practice this pranayama.
- People suffering from hernia, gastric ulcer, stroke, epilepsy or vertigo should also not practice Bhastrika pranayama.

- Bhastrika pranayama should be practiced under guidance of a trained yoga expert by people suffering from lung diseases such as asthma and bronchitis. Also inform their physician.
- People who have tuberculosis or are recovering from it are advised to practice it under guidance of a trained yoga expert.
- One must be aware of the abdominal breathing technique before attempting to practice advanced version of Bhastrika pranayama or even bhastrika also.
- Advanced practitioners can combine moola bandha and jalandhara bandha once they have mastered Bhastrika pranayama for best results. Both the nostrils must be clear while practicing bhastrika pranayama.

Anuloma Pranayama

Anulom Vilom (Alternate Nostril Breathing) is one of the most effective pranayamas to purify your body and mind. It cures the tri-dosas or impurities i.e. Vata, Pitta, and Kapha and is very useful in releasing stress and anxiety. In developing yoga practice, learning breath control exercises play an important role. According to Patanjali Yoga Sutras, pranayama is one of the classical eight limbs of Yoga. It helps to cleanse, balance, purify your life force or prana and helps you to stay healthy in mind, body, and spirit. This breathing practice is also called Nadi Shodhan pranayama as this clears your blocked energy channels.

In this breathing practice, inhalation (Puraka), retention (Kumbhaka) and exhalation (Rechaka) are used. This can be practised with or without Kumbhaka. Beginners should practice without Kumbhaka and with regular practice, they should bring that into their practice.

In Anulom Vilom pranayama, breathing can be done only through one nostril which is alternated, the other nostril is closed using the fingers. The thumb finger is used to close the right nostril and the ring finger is used to close the left nostril.

Steps of Anulom Vilom Pranayam

Sit on a mat on the floor. Cross your legs into the padmasana pose. If you cannot fold your knees completely, bend them as much as you can.

Those who have arthritis can sit on a wooden chair with a straight back. Now place one hand with the palms facing the ceiling. Place the thumb of your other hand on one nostril and fold the index finger. Keep the ring finger extended so that it can be used to close the other nostril.

Do not lift your elbow too high, your hand will get fatigued after a while. Leave it loose and by your side. Now inhale deeply through one nostril while keeping the other one closed with your finger. Now, open the other nostril and close the one you breathed in and exhale. This is one cycle.

To start the next cycle, breathe in through the same nostril that you exhaled out of and repeat the process. Practice this asana for about three minutes initially gradually increasing the amount of time to 15 to 20 minutes.

The left nostril represents the energy of the moon that symbolizes peace and tranquil and therefore, has a cooling effect. If you must purify the different Nadis or channels of the body, you must begin anulom vilom pranayama with the left nostril and exhale with the right. This is referred to as "one cycle". Start the second cycle by inhaling with the right nostril and exhaling with the left.

Repeat the cycles steadily in the beginning i.e. till your body has become strong. As the days pass, increase the number of cycles and reach the optimum level gradually. Once you have achieved the strength to practice the cycles for a longer duration, inhale with as much force as you can and then exhale with the same intensity. While you are repeating this pranayama, repeat "OM" in your mind. This meditation technique is helpful in uniting the body with spiritual powers to help reap the maximum benefits of anulom vilom possible.

Pace of Breathing: While doing this exercise, no breathing sound should be audible. The speed of inhalation and exhalation should be so gentle that even a small wad of cotton placed near the nostrils would not move. Ensure that the time taken during rechak or exhalation is double the time taken during purak or inhalation.

Practice: Close your eyes during pranayam. Imagine that your Sushumna nadi is being awakened by the friction of the Idaa and Pingla nadis and that energy is flowing right from the Muladhar Chakra or base chakra to the Shasraar Chakra or crown chakra. Believe that your entire body is being cleansed and made healthy.

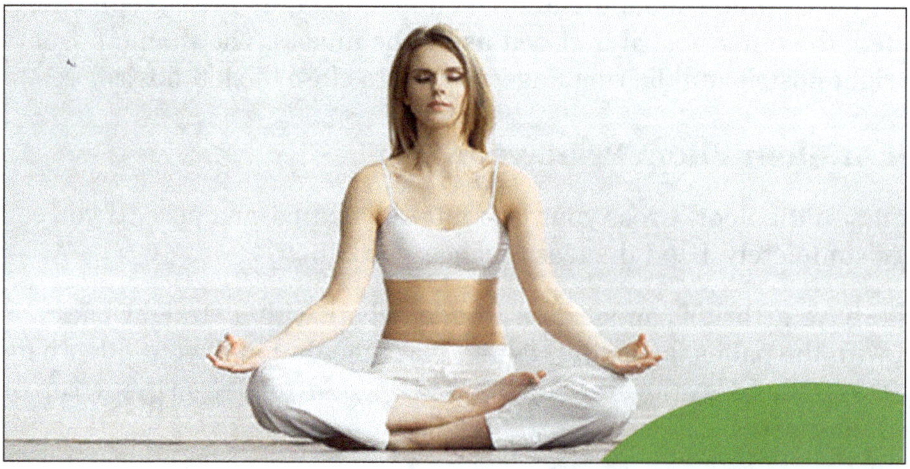

Benefits of Anulom Vilom Pranayam

Not just Yogis know anulom vilom pranayama benefits. Scientists also have discovered through a research that the nasal cycle corresponds with brain function. The electrical activity of the brain was found to be greater on the side opposite the less congested nostril. The right side of the brain controls creative activity, while the left side controls logical verbal activity.

The research showed that when the left nostril was less obstructed, the right side of the brain was predominant. Test subjects were indeed found to do better on creative tests. Similarly when the right nostril was less obstructed the left side of the brain was predominant. Test subjects did better on verbal skills.

Not just the brain, practising of anulom vilom pranayam regularly purifies the different channels of the body, making it healthy, strong and lustrous.

It cures all the diseases that occur due to the disturbance of the 'Vata Dosha'. These include rheumatism, gout, diseases that are related to the reproductive organs, and cold.

- The three doshas of Vata, Kapha and Pitta are also regularised with regular practice of anulom vilom pranayam.
- Blood pressure and diabetes can be cured completely with the regular and dedicated practice of this pranayam.
- Diseases of the muscular system are cured and are beneficial in arthritis, flatulence and varicose veins, acidity and sinusitis.
- Thinking becomes positive and you learn to overcome tension, anger, worry and forgetfulness, anxiety, uneasiness, high blood pressure, migraine and lack of sleep.
- Concentration, patience, resoluteness, decision-making ability and creativity also increase as advantages of anulom vilom pranayam.
- Increases oxygen supply throughout the body, making one feel calm and peaceful.
- Relieves stress , fever, eye concerns and ear issues.
- Improves blood circulation.
- Treats migraine, blockages in the arteries of the heart and chronic sinus problems.
- Transforms negative thoughts to positive.
- Controls obesity.

- Streamlines metabolism.
- Treats conditions of constipation, gastric, acidity, allergic problems, asthma, diabetes , gastric problems and snoring.

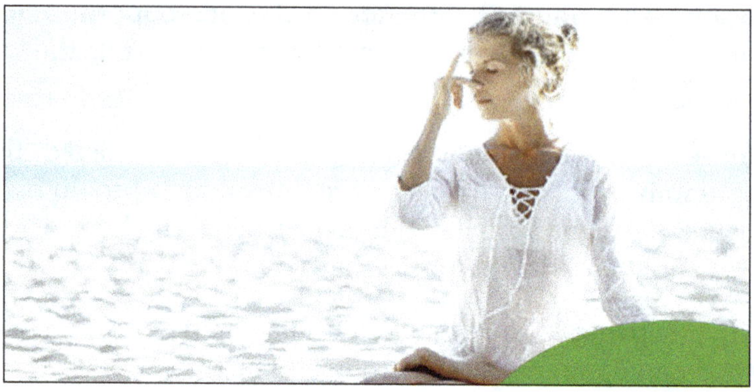

Best Time to Practice Anulom Vilom Pranayam

Pranayama or breathing exercise can be a great way to start your day. Early morning is the best time to practice and reap anulom vilom pranayama benefits, especially outside where you can find fresh air. It is recommended to do breathing exercises on an empty stomach.

Tip: To do pranayama sit facing east or north in a comfortable cross legged position on a yoga mat. Make sure your head, neck and chest are in a straight line and keep your spine stretched. Pranayama should not be performed within an hour of eating, bathing or sexual activity without at least an hour gap.

Precautions

- If you feel little bit of discomfort then you can reduce the ratio of breathing.
- Under No circumstances the proportion of the breathing should be forced.
- Practitioner should NEVER cross his body stamina and should never try over practice to get benefits earlier, as it may cause fatigue or giddiness.
- People who have undergone abdominal surgeries, heart surgeries, brain surgeries should consult the medical expert or consultant.
- Please do not rush to increase the proportions, as it will not help, but trying to practice easy ratio (4:6 seconds) for little more time may help.
- Initially one should start slowly by inhalation in 3 sec and exhalation in 3 sec. Slowly you an increase it to 4 : 4 sec then 3 : 6 sec and then 4 : 8 sec.
- The practice can be up to 5 minutes initially but slowly one can increase it to 15 minutes safely.

- be patient and practice regularly and constantly. Increase practice gradually after the body gains more stamina within few days.
- This is very good breathing exercise for women during pregnancy but over straining must be avoided.

Benefits

There are a lot of things that you are probably doing wrong, right from consuming excessive junk, having a wrong sleeping pattern to traveling in a dusty environment. This Pranayam can help you to deal with a lot of complications that arise from such a hectic lifestyle. Here is how anulom vilom pranayam benefits you:

- It helps you deal with problems like obesity, high blood pressure, asthma and many breathing problems increasing due to this.
- Daily exercise can lower the risk of these problems. Also, home therapy has lesser side effects as compared to medication therapy.
- Can help you deal with heart-related problems as well.

Many practitioners also use this form of yoga to treat problems like a migraine and sinus:

1. Anulom Vilom Pranayam doesn't just help you deal with diseases – there are a lot of other benefits too that help you lead a better life.

2. Skin: Direct exposure to the sun can damage your skin and the dust trapped in the air covers the skin making it dull. Yoga not only enhances the glow and makes it beautiful but also tighten the skin making it look younger.

3. Digestion: Digestive problems affect our stomach as well as skin and mind. Yoga regulates the digestive system and filters the internal organs keeping it clean and healthy.

4. Mental problems: Are depression and anxiety ruling your mind? Whether it's the next career step that you are worried about or something else, stress can be difficult to alleviate. Irregular sleeping patterns mean that you can't pull through the day easily – you would just be too tired. Yoga lowers stress level and relaxes your mind, helping you feel refreshed.

5. Reversing Your Heart Disease: If you're suffering from a heart ailment, including blockages in the arteries, Anulom Vilom Pranayam can help. The regular breathing exercise helps to reduce the blockage. The pace of breathing and regular inhalation means that you have a better blood circulation within the body, which helps the heart to pump properly.

Anulom Vilom Pranayam for Weight loss

That's not all, one of its major benefit is its ability to help you lose weight apart from helping achieve a calm and clear mind:

- Lesser time required: Doing 15-20 minutes of Anulom Vilom regularly helps a lot to lose weight.
- Easy: Alike power yoga and other difficult asanas, this pranayam is easy and compatible for people especially beginners. This is a must have tool if you are targeting overall wellness along with sustainable weight loss.
- Improves metabolism: It increases capacity which makes other exercises perform with less difficulty. Better metabolism means better fat burning capacity.
- Balances hormones: Women facing PCOD problems generally gain weight. It helps in balancing hormones, reducing weight and increase stamina.

Anulom Vilom Pranayama Side Effects

Everything that we do for our well being must be done in a well-balanced manner. Nothing can be done without having a control over it. Because it is rightly said that an excess of anything can be dangerous. It is like poison! So, here is what you need to know about the Anulom Vilom Pranayama side effects.

1. It is not a Medicine

One of the major side effects of Anulom Vilom is that it simply cannot be treated as a medicine to cure deadly illnesses. Professional aid has to be taken in case of critical problems.

2. Can Affect Mentally and Physically

Excessively practicing Anulom Vilom Pranayama affects your mental health to a cause a lifelong impact. And in case you are already dealing with any mental or physical ailments, do consult your physician to ensure safety.

3. Troubles after Meals

If you are practicing Anulom Vilom Pranayama right after your meals, you are inviting troubles for yourself. Practice the same early in the morning on an empty stomach (a little water does no harm) or least 4-5 hours post lunch.

4. Causes you to Inhale Bacteria

For people who breathe at a much faster rate may have to face difficulties at times. You are always at the risk of inhaling bacteria and other damaging viruses. So, these toxic elements in the environment can easily cause harm to the system over the time.

5. Makes you even Weaker

People who are physically weaker and are also afflicted with anemia must try this exercise with utmost care and if necessary, then only under supervision or after taking medical assistance. Make sure to not exceed the count of 4 for each breath that you inhale as well as exhale. Otherwise, you are always at risk of facing critical health issues.

6. Dangerous for Beginners

Although there's no problem with doing Anulom Vilom Pranayam, if you are a first-timer and you have simply seen or heard the steps of doing the exercise, then it is suggested to consult an expert. Usually, we understand something but interpret and practice it in some other way, which can actually be dangerous.

7. Causes Discomforts

Other the other Anulom Vilom Pranayama side effects are lethargy, dizziness, headache, unstable thought process, vomiting sensations, uneasiness, indigestion, mild depression, drying of mouth, lowering immunity, blurred vision and/or backache.

These are just a few Anulom Vilom Pranayam side effects and discomforts but if there's no control over it, circumstances can worsen.

Bhramari Pranayama

Bhramari Pranayama is made from the hindi word "Bhramar" (मधुमक्खी in Indian language) which means bumble Bee and the meaning of Pranayama is breathing technique so it can also called 'bee breath'. Bhraamri (Bee Breath) could be a terribly effective Pranayama (breathing exercise) for meditation. Activity of this respiratory exercise helps to induce a chilled impact on the mind rapidly. Bhramari Pranayama edges in reducing high vital sign, fatigue, and mental stress. Conjointly active this Pranayama for ear, nose, mouth, and eye issues will have a positive impact. This Pranayam is one of the great breathing exercises to release the mind of disquiet, anxiety or frustration and get rid of anger. It is a simple to do breathing technique and can be practiced anywhere at work or home, it is a instant option for de- stress yourself.

In Bhramari Pranayama the exhalation sound is very resembles to the humming sound of a bee, by this it is named as Bhramari pranayama. In this respiration process, your lips are purported to be shut, and you're purported to gently and swimmingly build a sound sort of a buzzing bee in your throat. The practice of Bhramari Pranayama is very helpful for making the breath smooth and quieting the mind too. You easily can feel the sound vibrations in your jaws, throat and face. This is simple and can be done by any age group of people.

Practice for Bhramari

Choose a comfortable sitting position. If you are able, it is best to sit cross-legged on the floor with a cushion or blanket to comfortably elevate the hips. Alternatively, you may choose to sit toward the front of a chair, with your feet flat on the floor. Allow the spine to lengthen so that the back, neck, and head are erect. Gently close the lips, keeping the teeth slightly apart, and bring the tip of your tongue to the space behind the upper front teeth. Maintain this position of the mouth throughout the practice, frequently checking to ensure that the jaw remains relaxed. Then, close each ear with the thumbs, place the index fingers at the midpoint of the forehead—just above the eyebrows—and reach the middle, ring, and pinky fingers across the eyes so that the tips of these fingers press very gently against the bridge of the nose.

To begin, take a long, deep breath in through the nostrils, bringing the breath all the way into the belly. Drop the chin to the chest and begin to exhale slowly, making a steady, low-pitched 'hmmm' sound at the back of the throat—like the humming of a bee. Focus on making the sound soft, smooth, and steady. The positioning of the tongue allows the vibration to better resonate throughout the head, affecting the tissues of the brain. Keep the body completely still and bring your awareness to the center of the head—to ajna chakra—letting the sound fill the head and spread to the body. Merge with the sound and allow the vibration to permeate your entire being. At the end of the exhalation, slowly straighten your neck as you inhale again through the nostrils to repeat the process. Begin with seven repetitions. You may either continue with seven repetitions, or you may add one repetition per week, slowly building up to a total of seventeen repetitions.

After the final exhalation, allow your breath to return to normal and observe any changes that have occurred. How do you feel physically, mentally, emotionally, and spiritually? What energetic shifts do you notice as a result of this practice? Where do you notice sensation in your body and how is it different from when you started? When you are ready, gently open your eyes, continuing to direct some of your awareness within. If it is morning, slowly stand and offer your full attention to the rest of your day; if it is evening, notice the vibrational calm that this practice has initiated in your body and try to maintain it as you prepare to retire for the night.

The above instructions are meant to provide a safe and general introduction to the practice of bhramari. Advanced practitioners sometimes add variations such as breath retention (khumbaka), muscular locks (bandhas), and may also hum on the inhalation—as in ujjayi pranayama. These additional techniques are best learned in person from a qualified teacher.

Bhramari (as with most pranayamas) is best practiced on an empty stomach. While it can be practiced at any time of day, bhramari is particularly potent in the early morning and late at night—when there are fewer distracting noises and our inner perception is most acute.

Precautions for doing Bhramari Pranayama

- Ensure that you are not putting your finger inside the ear but on the cartilage;
- Don't press the cartilage too hard. Gently press and release with the finger;
- While making the humming sound, keep your mouth closed;
- You can also do Bhramari pranayama with your fingers in the Shanmukhi Mudra;
- Do not put pressure on your face;
- Do not exceed the recommended repetitions of 3-4 times.

Contraindications

Once this pranayama is learnt correctly from a yoga teacher, anyone from a child to an elderly person can practice this pranayama. The only prerequisite is that this pranayama should be done on empty stomach.

Bahya Pranayama

The word Bahya is made from Sanskrit word Baahya which means outside or external.

Bahya Pranayama is one of the vital respiration exercises in which you have to forcibly breathe in (inhale), breath out and then hold the breath (retention). In this, the breathing is kept outside during the process so that's why this Pranayama is named as Baahya Pranayama. Meaning of Baahya is external and Pranayama means breathing technique so it is also called external Retention. Retention means holding the breath (Kumbhaka). 1:2:3 is the ratio of this Pranayama. The Ratio of 1:2:3 is meaning that breathes in takes one second, breathes out should be 2 seconds and holding the breath ought to be for three seconds.

Similarly, if breath in takes four seconds then breathes out ought to take eight seconds and holding the breath ought to be for twelve seconds that is nothing however 1:2:3.

Steps of Bahya pranayama:

- Sit in the padmasana (Lotus pose) close your eyes keep your spinal cord and head erect.
- Breathe in deeply (inhale).
- Then Exhale completely, evacuate your lungs as much as possible.

- After exhale hold your breath.
- Try to pull your stomach upward as much as you can, pull up the muscles in the area below the navel.

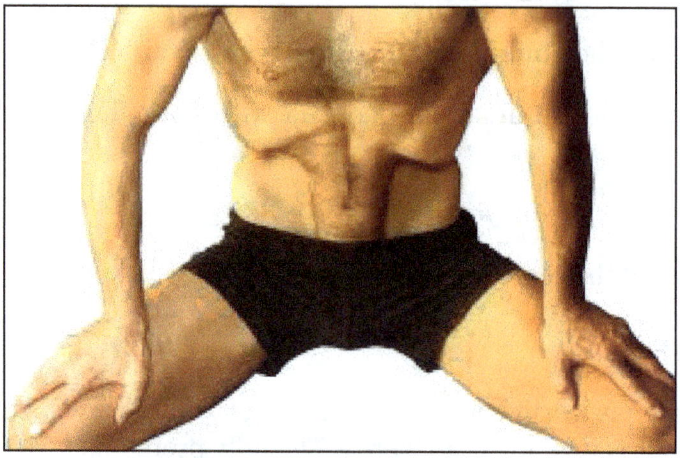

- After that move your head in down position so that your chin touches your chest.
- Hold this position for 5 to 10 seconds.
- Then relax and get back to starting position.
- If you have neck and back pain, do not move your head down. Just look straight.
- Repeat this process for five to ten times.

Benefits

1. It improves the digestive power and is beneficial in stomach ailments.
2. Constipation, Acidity, Gastric problem,Hernia cure completely.
3. Beneficial in problems related to constipation, piles, fissures, thyroid, throat, regenerative organs, uterus and urinary disorders, prostrate problems are also cured.
4. Problems related prostate get cure.
5. Cures problems related reproductive organs.
6. Good for diabetes as well.
7. Urine and sperm related problems get cure completely.
8. Mastering over it is rejuvenate.(Refresh, revitalize, renew).

9. Hernia is completely cured with regular practice.
10. It makes the intellect sharp and subtle.

Precaution

1. Heart patients should not practice bahya pranayama.
2. Patients with high blood pressure do not even think of attempting to practice bahya pranayama.
3. If a person has been living a normal blood pressure medication, that person after ten to twelve seconds doctor may external pranayama.
4. Bahya Pranayama should always be done on empty stomach.
5. Pregnant women should not practice Bahya Pranayama.
6. During Menstrual cycle (period time), the women should not bahya pranayama.
7. After holding your breath out, you will at least need 10 to 12 seconds to hold the above said three locks. Hence you must make sure that your body can stay at ease with your breath held for at least 10 to 12 seconds. Respect the ability of your body and decide to practice so that you don't cause any harm to your body by overdoing it.
8. It could harm you fatally if you attempt to practice it without having proper knowledge and practice to do it.

Important Things to Remember

Breathing exercise or Pranayama should practice on empty stomach, if you already had your meal then try to practice after 5-6 hours.

People suffering from heart diseases, high blood pressure, cervical colitis need to avoid doing this Bahya Pranayam.

Women should avoid practicing Bahya pranayama in the time of period.

Consult your doctor and yoga expert to avoid any unnecessary injury and to get the better results.

References

- 363-pranayama-and-its-yogic-importance, Ayurveda treatments, index: ayurvedatreatments.co.in, Retrieved 30,June 2020
- The-importance-of-pranayama-in-yoga-practice: yogawithsapna.com, Retrieved 10,July 2020

- Anulom-vilom-pranayama-side-effects: ayurvedum.com, Retrieved 30,May 2020
- Healing-Precautions-During-Anulom-Vilom-Pranayama: myguru.in, Retrieved 25,May 2020
- Bhramari-pranayama-bee-breath-steps-and-benefits: sarvyoga.com, Retrieved 31,March 2020
- Bhastrika-pranayama-the-bellows-breath: yogicwayoflife.com, Retrieved 30,March 2020
- Pranayama-in-yoga: yogiclogic.com, Retrieved 20,June 2020
- Benefits-anulom-vilom-pranayam-1331102533: onlymyhealth.com Retrieved 31, May 2020

6

Shatkarma: Yoga Cleansing Techniques

The set of practices within hatha yoga which aim at purifying the body in order to prepare a person for moksha, or liberation, is known as shatkarma. These practices include neti, dhauti, nauli, basti, kapalabhati and trataka. The topics elaborated in this chapter will help in gaining a better perspective about these purification techniques used in yoga.

Shatkarma is the Sanskrit term for one of the six yogic purification techniques (kriyas) as outlined in the "Hatha Yoga Pradipika." The purpose of these cleansing techniques is to keep the body strong, clean and healthy. They are said to remove toxins and anything blocking the flow of prana in the body.

Practicing shatkarmas internally purifies the body, which makes pranayama and meditation practice easier by preparing the body to perform these practices without distraction, discomfort or fatigue.

The shatkarmas should always be learned from and practiced under the supervision of an experienced teacher.

Those shatkarma which effect purification of the body are secret. They have manifold, wondrous results and are held in high esteem by eminent yogis. Yogic science gives as much importance to certain cleansing processes as it does to asana or pranayama. Without regular cleansing of the system one cannot gain maximum benefit from yoga practices. Without purification of the body one will not be ready for the higher practices of yoga.

Body cleansing is brought about by the practice of the shatkarmas or six purificatory techniques which are very important from the point of view of physical and mental health. These simple techniques are also highly valuable in healing internal disorders. There are six main groups of shatkarmas or yogic cleansers as follows:

1. Neti: nasal cleaning, including jala neti and sutra neti.
2. Dhauti: cleansing of the digestive tract.
3. Nauli: abdominal massage.
4. Basti: colon cleaning.
5. Kapalbhati: purification and vitalisation of the frontal lobes.

6. Trataka: blinkless gazing.

Each of these groups contains more than one practice, such as jala neti, vaman dhauti (or kunjal kriya), moola shodhana etc. They are all excellent practices designed to purify the whole body and bring about first-class health. They also bring clarity and harmony to the mind.

'Shatkarma' (sometimes known as Shatkriya) is a compound word consisting of two components: 'shat' meaning 'six' and 'karma' meaning 'art' or 'process'. The word 'kriya' or 'karma' is used in Hatha Yoga in a special technical sense regarding the techniques of cleaning. Although we have grouped them into six here, the 'Gherand Samhita' and 'Hatha Yoga Samhita' enumerate as many as twenty-one such practices, albeit under six broad headings. The 'Shatkarma Samgraha' describes no less than forty-six such processes, such as vamana, vireehana, gandusha, udgara, and raktasrava.

The 'Hatha Yoga Pradipika' however is the only authentic work which tends to limit itself exactly to six cleansing practice, 'Pranatoshani' refers to only five purificatory practices. Besides these works, a vernacular treatise, 'Bhakti Sagram' of Charana Das describes in detail the shatkarmas and in addition mentions four mere which it does not describe. Dhauti, basti, neti, trataka, nauli and kapalbhati are the six traditionally known processes.

The shatkarma affect and activate almost all of the vital systems in the body, especially the digestive, respiratory, circulatory and nervous systems. Every individual organ of importance, like the food pipe, stomach, colon, lungs, eyes and ears, receives equal attention. These purificatory processes are both preventive and curative.

The shatkarma are very powerful practices that can never be learned from books or taught by inexperienced people. Only these instructed by the guru can teach others. One may think that he has the capacity to teach but actually he may not have adequate experience or knowledge to guide ethers proficiently. This applies to the shatkarma in particular. If unqualified people teach them they are likely to make serious mistakes. Also, one can make mistakes if one practises them independently without the aid of a guru.

They are said to be 'secret' practices as one must be personally instructed how to perform them and how often, according to individual need. For this, a qualified and experienced teacher is essential. Those who sincerely want to learn the shatkarma will have to find a guru of hatha yoga, and they will have to search hard, for few teachers are expert in the shatkarma. There are three humours in the body:kapha(mucus),pita(bile), andvata (wind). In yoga and ayurveda they are calledtridasha. A balanced proportion of these three facilitates body functions, but if there is excess of one and shortage of another, ailments develop due to overheating or not enough heat in the body. So, before commencing pranayama, any imbalance in the doshas should be removed.

The effects of the shatkarma can be summed up in one word - purification. When the different systems of the body have been purified, the overall result is that energy can flow through the body freely. One's capacity to work, think, digest, taste, feel, experience, etc., increases and greater awareness develops. It is no wonder that the yogis who have attained perfection consider the shatkarma with great esteem.

General Benefits of Shatkarmas

1. Shatkarmas are very good to overcome from lot of diseases completely, so it's very effective in Yoga therapy.
2. The practise of shatkarma creates harmony in body and mind.
3. The different systems of the body are purifying this shatkarma practise, so the energy can flow through the body freely.
4. Its very good for general health, this increases the ones capacity to work, think, digest, taste, feel, experience, etc.

Neti

Neti is a type of yogic nasal cleansing exercise. It is one of six kriyas, or purification techniques also known as shatkarma, that are outlined in the "Hatha Yoga Pradipika." Neti kriya is designed to purify the nasal passages and bathe the sinuses.

The purpose of the kriyas is to keep the body strong, clean and healthy. They are said to remove toxins and anything blocking the flow of prana in the body. The kriyas are believed to prepare the body for yoga practice such as asanas, pranayama and meditation by eliminating physical distractions, discomfort and fatigue.

There are Three types of neti kriya:

1. Jala Neti,
2. Dugdha Neti,
3. Sutra Neti.

Jala Neti

Jala Neti is a yogic technique to clean your sinuses. Neti is one of the six purification methods in Hatha Yoga. The sinus cavities can get clogged with impurities which may cause infections, inflammations and headaches. The yogic text Hatha Yoga Pradeepika gives a simple method to keep your sinuses clean. The text gives six practices for cleansing the body and to prepare the body and mind for higher practices of Yoga. These are called Shatkarmas. One of them deals with Nasal hygiene and is called Neti. Nasal hygiene is extremely important as it is linked to many conditions like sinusitis, migraine, headaches, allergies and asthma. Neti is a very simple practice that can be done along with your daily routine, say immediately after brushing your teeth in the morning. It takes just a few minutes and helps to relieve many of the problems related to the nasal and sinus cavities.

To do Jala Neti (Neti using plain warm saline water), you need a Neti Pot, some salt and water. Neti pot is a small pot with a long spout on the side which is inserted into one of the nostrils during the practice. It can be made of copper, steel, ceramic or even plastic. It is available in most health stores that sell yoga products. Prepare salt water by mixing 1 table spoon of salt to one liter of warm water. The salt should be of the right proportion and the water should be slightly warm so that it does not irritate the tissues inside the nostrils. Neti practiced with water is called Jala Neti. Neti can also be done using milk and is then called Dugdha Neti.

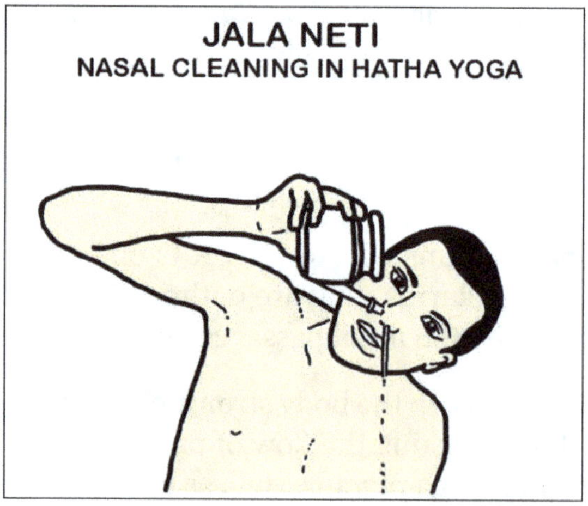

Practice for Jala Neti

1. Pour the salt water into the Neti pot and place the spout of the pot into one of the nostrils, say the left nostril. The cone at the end of the spout should to be placed inside the nostril.

2. Tilt your head gently and open your mouth (Breathing should be done through the mouth during the process). Adjust the tilt of your head up to a point where water starts flowing from your left nostril to the right nostril. Continue till the water in the pot is finished.

3. Fill the pot again with salt water and try the same procedure from the other nostril (say the right nostril).
4. You can repeat this process any number of times, depending on your need and time.

When you first start this practice, you may get irritations in the nose, sneezing, coughing, etc. which will disappear after few sessions.

For those with thick mucus conditions as well as those with running sinuses, the relief of sinus pressure can be felt within seconds. As well, the eustachian tubes (which are also dead end passages) receive exactly the same effects as the sinuses, that being – a drawing outwards of dirt and mucus. Hence Jala Neti is of great benefit for blockages and infections of the middle ear, by draining the tubes to relieve the pressure build up as well as removing germs. In a more detailed examination, it would also be seen that through the effect of osmosis and capillary action, the blood vessels of the nose are stimulated to cleanse as well.

The eyes are also beneficially affected by Neti. The tear ducts, which connect from the eyes into the nasal passages, get the same drawing out effect as the sinuses, and this results in a brighter, clearer sense of vision.

Neti removes all the dirt and bacteria filled mucus from within the nose.

It also helps to drain the sinus cavities. This in turn, will help to reprogramme the body's natural mechanisms against nasal infections such as hayfever, allergies, sinusitis and other upper respiratory complaints like sore throats and coughs, post nasal drip, inflammation of tonsils and adenoids.

It is beneficial for illnesses such as asthma and bronchitis as it reduces the tendency for mouth breathing by freeing the nostrils of mucus.

- It has a cooling and soothing effect on the brain by drawing out excessive heat, and is therefore beneficial for headaches, migraine, epilepsy, temper tantrums, hysteria, depression and general mental.
- Neti is of great benefit for problems associated with the eyes. It helps flush the tear ducts, encouraging clearer vision and gives a sparkle to the eyes.
- It can be beneficial for certain types of ear disorders such as middle ear infections, glue ear, tinitis.
- Neti improves sensitivity of the olfactory nerves, helping to restore lost sense of smell, and thereby benefits the relationship with taste and the digestive processes.
- It has subtle effects on the pineal and pituitary glands which control the

hormonal system. This has a harmonising effect on emotional behaviour.

- Neti affects the psychic centre known as Ajna Chakra which helps in awakening higher states of meditation.
- It helps to stimulate better powers of visualisation and concentration and gives a feeling of lightness and clarity to the mind.
- Neti is excellent for those trying to give up smoking. Since it reduces the tendency for mouth breathing, Neti re-sensitises the nose to the actual pollution of ingesting smoke, thereby de-programming the brain of the physical and psychological addiction.

Dugdha Neti

The technique is not half as hard as it appears. In fact, once mastered, which should take a day or two at most. You will be surprised at both, the technique and its results. Another version of Netis is using diluted milk, pre-warmed to body temperature, in place of water. It is particularly beneficial to those suffering from chronic nose bleeding or for those who find salt water irritating.

Steps

- A special "Neti Pot" is first filled with milk, pre-warmed to body temperature. Its spout is then inserted into one nostril.
- Place the cone into your nostril, sealing it inside with a few gentle twists. The position of your head is adjusted, slightly tilted, to allow the milk to flow out your other nostril.
- Breathe gently through your mouth, trying not to sniff or swallow while the milk is flowing through.

Benefits

Dugdha Neti help extract all the impurity and bacteria filled mucus from the nasal and sinus cavities.

This in turn, will help to restore the body's mechanisms to natural and increase its immunity to nasal allergies like hay fever, sinusitis and other respiratory conditions like sore throats, chronic coughs and colds, post nasal drips, adenoids and tonsillitis.

Caution

Remember, under no circumstances should you experience pain in the practice.

If you feel any pain, it either means you are inserting the catheter too fast, or that it entered the wrong way and is stalled against the nasal wall, unless there is otherwise some other genetic obstruction.

In which case, stop immediately, withdraw and reinsert the catheter carefully in another direction until you find a clear unimpeded passage.

Sutra Neti

Sutra Neti is a Hatha yoga technique to clean your nasal cavity. Sutra Neti is one of the six methods of purification or Shatkarma as given in the yogic text Hatha Yoga Pradeepika. There are various types of Neti practiced by Yogis including Jala Neti (with water), Dughda Neti (with Milk), Sutra Neti (with cotton string), etc. In Sutra Neti, a waxed cotton string is traditionally used to clean the nasal cavity.

In Sutra Neti, the waxed cotton string is inserted into the nose and then pulled out from the mouth. Then both ends are held with the hands and nasal cleaning is done by to and fro motion of the strings. Nowadays, a rubber catheter is used instead of the string as it is easily available in any medical store.

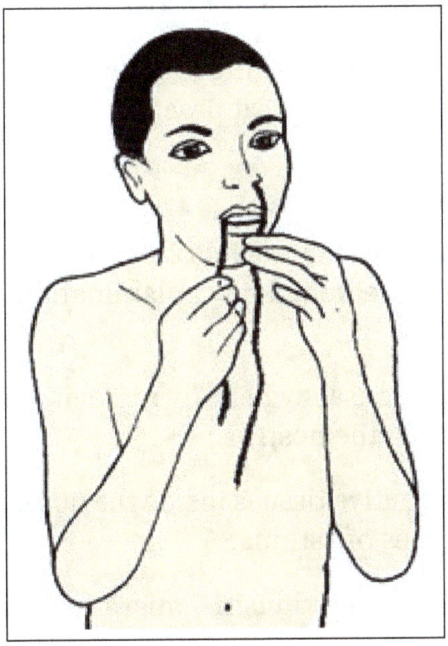

Steps of Sutra Neti

Sutra Neti should be learned from a qualified yoga instructor as it needs guidance in the beginning. This practice is ideally done in the early morning after brushing your teeth, though it can be practiced at any time of the day. Acquire a rubber catheter of size between 1 mm and 3 mm from any medical store. Select a size which you feel is comfortable for you to use, through trial and error or through expert advice.

- Take the rubber catheter in your hand and very gently insert the tube inside your left nostril. Take care not to rush it; do it very slowly as it can irritate the sensitive membrane inside the nostril. Many people have mild nasal septal deviations, which is more or less harmless. If the deviation is acute then one may feel a block while inserting the rubber tube. Seek expert guidance in such cases.

- Push the tube into your nostril upwards, till it hits the back of the throat. At this point the tube will bend and go down the throat. Continue inserting the catheter slowly.
- Open your mouth and use your middle and index fingers to grab the tube from inside your throat. This takes a little practice. Once you get the knack of it, you can do it with ease.
- Pull the tube out so that part of it is just outside the mouth. Never leave the other end of the tube, which you are holding with your other hand.
- Now using both hands move the tube in a massaging motion to clean the nostrils and throat.
- Repeat the procedure with the right nostril.
- After the practice is over, remove the catheter and clean it. Store the catheter in a clean place for another day's next practice.

Benefits of Sutra Neti

Sutra Neti has benefits similar to that of Jala Neti. The nasal cavities can get clogged with impurities which may cause infections, inflammations and headaches. Sutra Neti can give the following benefits:

- It helps to maintain the nasal hygiene by removing the dirt and bacteria trapped along with the mucus in the nostrils.
- It de-sensitizes the sensitive tissues inside the nose, which can alleviate rhinitis, allergies and some types of asthma.
- Several health problems like sinusitis, migraine, headaches, can be reduced by doing Neti.

Precautions to take while Performing Sutra Neti

This is thought to be a more advanced kriya than jal neti and it is generally recommended that you seek some guidance from an expert before attempting this on your own. It is also recommended that a good quality rubber tube be used for the purpose. It should be soft and comfortable; the prescribed thickness is about 4mm but to begin with an even thinner tube or sutra can be used. The thickness can be increased as one gets more proficient at Sutra Neti.

If there seems to be a persistent blockage in the nasal passage, don't force it; instead get medical attention. Ensure that the tube is kept clean and stored in a dry place to prevent bacteria buildup.

Dhauti

A strip of wet cloth, four angulas wide (3") and fifteen hands (1¼ metres) in length, is stoutly swallowed and, then taken out, as instructed by the guru. This is known as dhauti.

Dhauti is divided, into four parts. According to the "Gherand Samhita" they are called antar (internal) dhauti, danta (teeth) dhauti, hrid (cardiac) dhauti, and moola shodhana (rectal cleansing). The practice described in this verse is actually vastra dhauti. 'Vastra' means 'cloth', This practice must only be performed under expert guidance and in full accordance with the instructions given.

The cloth should be of finely woven cotton which is clean and new. Synthetic material should definitely not be used. The cloth must also be trimmed neatly so that no fraying takes place. It should he no wider than the tongue or it will fold as it passes down the throat, and should be at least one meter and no more than a meter and a half in length.

Technique

Wash, rinse and boil the cloth well - keep it in a container of warm water while you are practising -squat with the heels on the ground and buttocks off the ground or resting - on a brick or something of the same height -relax the body - keep the cloth spread and not folded as you use it - spread one end over the tongue and start swallowing the cloth -if it catches in the throat and will not pass down, take a sip of warm water, but do not drink a large quantity - the stomach is to be filled with the cloth and not with water - the cloth tends to stick in the lowest point of the throat, so keep swallowing it and resist the urge to vomit - once (he cloth passes a little further down the oesophagus the problem will end -when two-thirds of the cloth have been swallowed, leave the remaining few inches hanging out of the mouth and stand up ready to practise nauli - the cloth can be left in the stomach for five to twenty minutes but no longer - practise dakshina (right) and vama (left) nauli; then rotations and madhyama nauli - five to ten minutes is sufficient time to clean the stomach - sit again in the squatting position and remove the cloth.

Vatsara Dhauti

Vatsara dhauti is performed by breathing in slowly through the mouth in kaki mudra and then swallowing the air into the stomach while expanding the abdomen. It can be done up to ten times or until the stomach is fully expanded. Then the air should be passed through the large intestine. To do this it is helpful to assume an inverted posture. Pashinee mudra is best. The air should then pass out of the anus easily.

Varisara Dhauti

Varisara dhauti is more commonly known today as shankhaprakshalana. In this practice you drink a total of sixteen glasses of warm salty water and evacuate it through the bowels. First you drink two glasses and perform a series of five specific asanas: tadasana, tiryaka tadasana, kati chakrasana, tiryaka bhujangasana and udarakarshan asana. After every two glasses the asanas should be performed until the water starts flowing out of the anus. Once clear water starts coming through, you will know that the stomach and intestines are perfectly clean and you can stop the practice.

Forty-five minutes after completing the practice, a saltless liquid mixture of cooked rice, mung dal, and ghee has to be eaten until the stomach is completely full. There are dietary restrictions to be observed for the minimum period of one week after the practice, and as it is a major cleansing operation, it must be done under expert guidance.

Laghoo Shankhaprakshalana

This is a shortened form of shankhaprakshalana. 'Laghoo' means 'short'. In this practice only six glasses of warm saline water are taken. After every two glasses the same series of asanas are to be performed as in 'poorna' (full) shankhaprakshalana.

The "Hatharatnaveli" mentions the use of jaggery water or milk water (1:5) instead of salt water. There are also various other herbs and juices which can be used, such as a few drops of lemon, onion or garlic. Laghoo shankhaprakshalana could be done with carrot or celery juice. Though not compulsory, we recommend that the practices of first kunjal kriya, and then jala neti be done immediately after completing shankhaprakshalana. This gives the best possible cleansing to the entire digestive tract.

Vahnisara Dhauti

Vahnisura dhauti, also known as agnisara kriya is a practice which involves moving the 'fire' in the body. 'Vahni' and 'agni' mean 'fire'. 'Sar' means 'essence'. This 'essence of fire' is located in the navel region. On a physical level, the practice involves conscious movement of the abdominal muscles and organs which creates internal heat. The practice is very useful as a preparation for kapalbhati and bhastrika pranayama.

Simple Form

Sit in vajrasana - keep the toes together and separate the knees as far as possible

- place the hands on the knees and keep the arms straight - lean forward slightly - open the mouth and extend the tongue outside - breathe rapidly in and out while simultaneously expanding and contracting the abdomen - the respiration should be in harmony with the movement of the abdomen and should resemble the panting) of a dog - breathe in and out up to 25 times - advanced practitioners can perform 50 - 100 breaths.

Advanced Form

Exhale as deeply as possible - perform jalandhara bandha (chin lock) - rapidly expand and contract the abdominal muscles for as long as you are able to retain the breath. For both forms the standing position can be used.

Benefits of Vahnisara Dhauti

This practice massages all the abdominal nerves, strengthens the muscles and stimulates the associated nerves, encouraging the best possible functioning of these organs. It promotes the correct secretion of digestive juices and thereby allows optimum assimilation of nutrients. It prevents and removes various digestive maladies such as constipation, indigestion, hyper - acidity, hypo-acidity, flatulence, constipation and sluggish liver.

Danta Dhauti

Danta dhauti is the cleaning of the teeth with a special stick, usually of neem or babool. A toothbrush and paste can also be used. It includes jihva dhauti-cleaning the tongue by rubbing it with the joined first finger and thumb in a downward motion, and then squeezing it, karna dhauti- cleaning the ears with the middle finger and nothing smaller, kapalrandhra - cleaning the upper back portion of the palate, chakshu dhauti -bathing the eyes with tepid saline water or urine.

Hrid Dhauti

The word 'hrid' means 'heart' or the chest region, and these practices are concerned with purifying this region of the body. The techniques are divided into three - Vastra dhauti, which has already been described, danda dhauti, and vaman dhauti.

Danda dhauti: This is the method of cleaning the oesophagus, the food pipe, from the throat to the stomach, by inserting a specially prepared stick. The stick is usually the soft core of a banana tree stem, being about half an inch in diameter and two feet long. The stem is carefully inserted down the throat until the end of it reaches the stomach. Then it is slowly removed. It should not be attempted under any circumstances without expert guidance. It removes mucus, phlegm, acidity and general impurities from the oesophagus.

Vaman dhauti or vyaghra kriya: This is the second practice of hrid dhauti. 'Vaman' is 'to vomit' 'vyaghra' means 'tiger'. Just as a tiger regurgitates its food a couple of hours after eating; in this practice you vomit the food from the stomach three hours after a meal. If it is difficult you can drink a glass or two of warm saline water and then tickle the back of the throat with the first two fingers to induce vomiting. Traditionally, after performing this practice, a sweet milk rice pudding should be eaten.

Kunjal kriya: is almost identical to vyaghra kriya, except that it is performed on an empty stomach. You drink four to six glasses of warm saline water and then vomit it out. There are no dietary restrictions afterwards.

Moola shodhana: is done by inserting the middle finger into the rectum and rotating it clockwise, then anticlockwise. Make sure the fingernail is cut short, and if necessary, you can put some non irritating oil on the finger to lubricate the anus. The "Gherand Samhita" also recommends the use of a turmeric root instead of the finger, and starting by sitting in utkatasana.

Bahiskrita dhauti: This is a very difficult practice unless you are an advanced hatha yogi. It involves standing navel deep in clean water, pushing the rectum out and washing it in the hands. The "Gherand Samhita" states, "It is not easily available even to the gods".

Benefits of the Dhauti Series

The 'Hatha Yoga Pradipika' states, "There is no doubt that cough, asthma, diseases of the spleen, leprosy and twenty kinds of diseases caused by excess mucus are destroyed through the effect of dhauti karma.' The combination of all the practices of dhauti cleans the entire digestive tract and respiratory tract. It removes excess and old bile, mucus and toxins, and restores the natural balance of the body's chemical composition, thus alleviating ailments caused by such imbalances.

The various practices help remove infectious bacteria from the mouth, nose, eyes, ears, throat, stomach, intestines and anus. The results are a reduction of excess fatty tissue and relief from flatulence, constipation, poor digestion and loss of appetite. Dhauti is even said to cure leprosy. Although this disease is not prevalent in many countries today, the point is that even such insidious diseases can be alleviated through this powerful practice.

The "Gherand Samhita" states that dhauti can cure abdominal ailments and fever, of course it is not advisable to practise dhauti during a fever or acute visceral infection- However, if it is practised after recuperation it will prevent recurrence of the problem. There are certain conditions in which antar dhauti must not be practised. These are: stomach or intestinal ulcers, hernia, heart disease, and high blood pressure.

Nauli

Nauli or Nauli Kriya is a technique for abdominal massage in Hatha Yoga. Benefits of Nauli are tremendous. It is one of the six purification methods or Shatkarma in Hatha Yoga. Nauli practitioners can maintain good health and vitality. But mastering this technique is not easy for beginners. It may take anything from three months to one year to perfect it depending on your body condition, your zeal and your effort.

Nauli is a powerful technique which massages all the organs in the abdomen – the stomach, the liver, spleen, urinary bladder, pancreas, gall bladder and the intestines. This helps to maintain perfect health of the lower organs.

The key to perfecting Nauli is the ability to isolate the muscles called rectus abdominis muscle (or the "abs" muscle) in the abdomen. These muscles are found on either side of the abdomen, running vertically and parallel all the way from the lower ribs on the top to the pubic region at the bottom.

There are three basic practices in Nauli. When this muscle is isolated to the left it is called Vama Nauli and when it is isolated to the right it is called Dakshina Nauli. When both the left and right muscles are concentrated to the center, it is called Madhya Nauli. Apart from these, rotation of the muscles is also practiced.

Nauli must be learned in the presence of a qualified yoga instructor. The best time to do the practice is early morning when the stomach and the bowels are empty. After a heavy meal, one should wait for at least 5 to 6 hours before attempting this practice. Do not overdo the practice as it may cause indigestion and loose motion. In such cases, discontinue the practice for few days and take guidance from a yoga expert.

The Four Steps of Nauli

The practice of nauli essentially involves four movements:

- Uddiyana bandha: This is an abdominal lock where you empty out your lungs and pull your stomach in and upward beneath your rib cage.
- Madhyana nauli (central nauli): Where you isolate and contract the abdominal muscles in the center.
- Vama nauli (left side nauli): Where you isolate and contract muscles on the left side of the abdomen.
- Daksina nauli (right side nauli): Where you isolate and contract muscles on the right side of the abdomen.

Uddiyana Bandha

1. Stand with your feet apart so that they extend a little more than the width of your hip. Now bend your knees a bit and place your hands on your thighs right above the knees.
2. Exhale completely so that all the air is pushed out. Remember to keep your stomach relaxed after you exhale.
3. With your breath exhaled, raise up your rib cage and pull the area under the navel up and inward, curving it toward your spine. Your lower back will round a bit and your pelvis will tuck under when you do this. Hold this position for a bit, say, a few seconds.
4. Release the position and inhale slowly through the nose. If you find yourself gasping for breath, you've held the position for too long.
5. Once you're comfortable with the uddiyana bandha, you can try doing uddiyana bandha contractions. This involves going in and out of the bandha without inhaling – that is, repeating and releasing the position described in step 3 without inhaling. In the beginning, you may find yourself getting out of breath pretty soon. With repeated practice, you may be able to do 5 to 10 contractions without inhaling.

Steps for Nauli

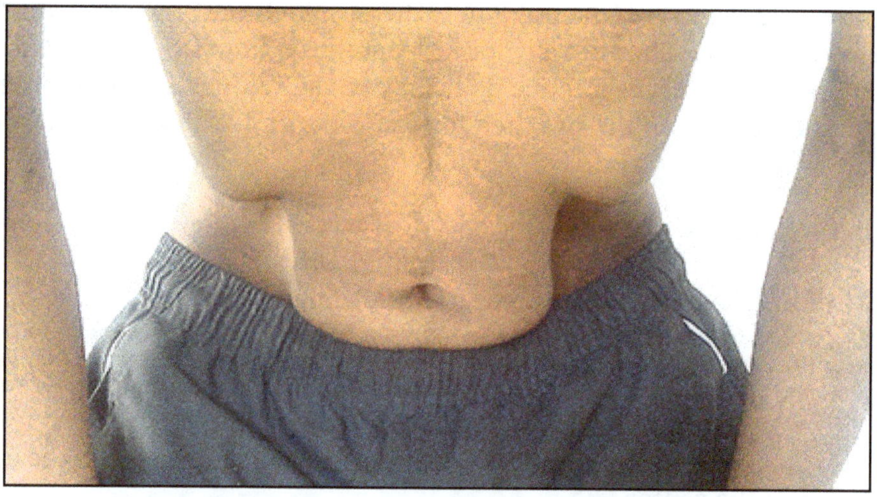

1. Stand with feet apart, knees bent and hands holding the thighs.
2. Take a deep breath and then force the breath out with a hissing sound.
3. Contract the belly inwards and upwards (towards the sternum). This is called Uddiyana Bandha. This is the base position for performing all the Nauli kriyas.

4. Hold the breath and try to isolate the two 'abs' muscles (or rectus abdominis muscles) and force them towards the center. There is no breathing involved. The breath is stopped with the air taken out of the lungs (also called Bahya Kumbhaka in Yoga). This takes bit of effort in the beginning. The main difficulty is in isolating the rectus abdominis muscles. Then you have to concentrate and position it in the center for at least few seconds. This comes with practice.

5. Now breathe in and release the position. Come to a fully standing position. Take a few deep natural breaths before trying again.

6. Try this few times according to your capacity.

7. Perfecting this may take from three months to a year for a beginner. Have patience. Once you master it, the benefits are great.

Steps for Vama Nauli

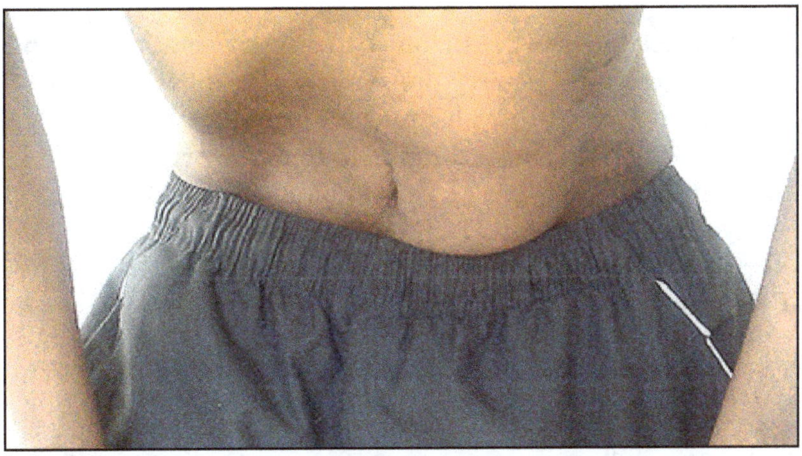

Take the same stance as in the earlier practice. Follow the steps 1 – 3 as mentioned in the Madhya Nauli practice.

1. Once you forcefully breathe out and perform Bahya Kumbhaka, get ready to do Vama Nauli.

2. In Vama Nauli only the left rectus abdominis muscles are isolated and pushed to the front. This will form a cavity in the right side and a muscle protrusion on the left side. Maintain this position for few seconds.

3. Breathe in and release the position and come to a standing position.

4. Take few deep breaths and repeat the process.

Steps for Dakshina Nauli

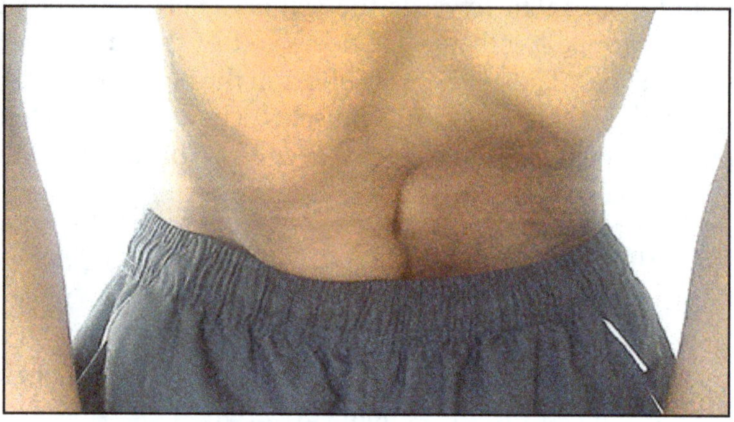

1. The procedure is same as the earlier practice of Vama Nauli.
2. The difference is instead of isolating the left abdominis muscles, the right abdominis muscles are flexed and isolated.

After mastering the three types of Nauli, one can also try rotating the abdominis muscles in the clockwise direction. Also try the same in the anti-clockwise direction. This looks like a churning motion of the 'abs' muscles from the left to right and from the right to left. This is a very powerful technique to tone the organs of the abdomen. The stomach, the intestines, spleen, liver, kidneys, pancreas, etc. get a good massage. If practiced regularly, this ensures good health of all these organs.

Beneficial Effects

1. The liver, one of the most important organs of the body will benefit of a stronger internal circulation and its functioning will be better.
2. The bile is quite well massaged during the practice of this technique. The practice of NAULI may also make the eventual stones move, generating their expulsion in quite a number of cases.
3. The pancreas will benefit by the practice of NAULI as well. Even if this technique cannot cure diabetes, it may nevertheless ensure a correct function of this gland, including the insulin-producer Langerhans isles.
4. Owing to the profound inhalations and exhalations, as well as to the void created in the thoraces while retaining your breath, NAULI contributes to regaining or maintaining the elasticity of your lungs.
5. Through the periodicity of pressure during the practice of this technique, the heart is also profoundly massaged. Thus, NAULI constitutes one of the best protections against heart attack. Once you fully master this technique, you will

also have your breath under control and you may even feel in your mouth an unusual flavour.

6. NAULI makes the practitioner immune to diseases such as: hernia, appendicitis, ulcer, indigestion, constipation, etc.

The fundamental yogic treatise the HATHA YOGA PRADIPIKA asserts:

"Sitting on the toes with heels raised above the ground, and the palms resting on the ground, and in this bent posture the belly is moved forcibly from left to right, just as in vomiting. This is called by adepts the Nauli Karma.

It removes dyspepsia, increases appetite and digestion, and is like the goddess of creation, and causes all happiness. It dries up all the disorders. This is an excellent exercise in Hatha Yoga."

Basti

Sitting in utkatasana, naval deep in water, insert a tube in the anus and contract the anus. This cleansing with water is called basti karma.

The Sanskrit word 'basti' (written as 'vasti' or 'wasti') is a general word that relates to anything pertaining to the lower abdomen, belly, pelvis and bladder. The practice of basti karma is a process of cleaning the lower abdomen, especially the colon. The word 'sthala' means 'ground'. Sthala basti is a practice where one stands on dry ground, i.e., one sucks air into the anus instead of water- The technique is also called 'sushka basti', 'sushka' meaning 'dry'. Another name for air basti is vata basti where the word 'vata' means 'air'. It is the practice which cleans the colon by sucking air into the body. In this practice, no external aid in the form of a catheter or tube is to be used.

The word 'jala' means 'water'. Jala basti is the practice whereby one sucks water into the anus. It is also called 'vati basti' which also means water. Vari basti is the process of cleaning the colon with water. The method for both sthala and jala basti is exactly the same, the only difference being that sthala basti is practised in air and jala basti in water. In this practice, unlike sthala basti, hatha yoga permits the use of a catheter tube.

Technique

Jala Basti

If a river is not available, the practice can be done over a bucket or basin of water. Beginners will have to start by inserting a 0.8cm catheter into the rectum. Traditionally, a bamboo tube was used. Plastic tubing or a catheter are suitable but organic material is always preferable. The tube should be at least 13-15cms long, preferably smooth and hollow. Lubricate it with beeswax or a non-irritating oil such as vaseline or ghee.

Insert 4cms of the tube into the anal passage or as much as possible, then squat over the bucket or basin in utkatasana. Exhale and perform uddiyana bandha. If the water is not sucked up through the tube into the bowel, then do madhyama nauli and hold. If the water is still not sucked up do vama, or dakshina nauli. When you can no longer hold kumbhaka, remove the catheter or tube without exhaling. Then stand up and exhale slowly through the nose. When you expel the water it is best to squat over the toilet because stool in the lower intestine will also come out. If the catheter is not removed before exhaling, the water will pass out and the tube may get blocked by pieces of stool.

After much practice the catheter will not be necessary as you will be able to suck water into the bowel directly, but that is a very advanced stage which may take years to perfect. When practising without the catheter you have to push the rectum out as far as possible, then draw it in with uddiyana. First you open the sphincter muscles with the fingers, perform uddiyana and remove the hand. Maintain kumbhaka for as long as possible and then slowly exhale.

After the practice, make sure all the water is expelled. Then lie in shavasan on a blanket. Slowly assume pashinee mudra, placing the knees beside the ears and balancing or the backs of the shoulders, hands clasped behind the back of the knees. This releases air from the bowel and induces a bowel action if there is any water remaining.

Come out of the position slowly and lie in shavasana again. Then fold the knees to the chest, hold them and slowly rock from side to side, or rock with the arms stretched out to the sides at shoulder level. Lie in shavasana again, and when you are ready, perform bhujangasana slowly 3-5 times. This exerts pressure on the lower intestines and releases any remaining water or air. Those who are able should perform mayurasana. Pashinee mudra is the most suitable counter-pose.

It is extremely important that the water used in basti is perfectly clean and neither too hot nor too cold. In cold weather lukewarm water should be used. It is not necessary to add salt to the water but the catheter must be sterilised before and after use. Basti car be done in warm or hot weather, especially if you are also doing intense pranayama and bandhas. Basti generates energy but also removes heat from the system. It must not be done during cloudy, rainy, windy or stormy weather.

Sthala Basti

Sthala or dry basti is performed while lying on the back. Assume Vipareeta karani mudra but position the back at a 60° angle to the floor. Then bring the knees down to the chest. Push the sphincter muscles out and in, so air is sucked into the bowel. This is not an easy practice and jala basti has to be perfected first. Sthala basti can also be practised in pashinee mudra or paschimottanasana, performing ashwini mudra. Uddiyana may also be required in the beginning. In paschimottanasana it is not easy to suck in air as there is pressure on the anus, so it is best to start in an inverted asana. The 'Hatharatnavali' says "After practising basti, do not take food for three ghatis.

Benefits

According to the 'Hatha Yoga Pradipika', 'Enlargement of the glands and spleen and all diseases arising from excess wind, bile and mucus are eliminated from the body through the practice of basti.' With reference to jala basti it states, "By practising jala basti the appetite increases, the body glows, excess doshas are destroyed and the dhatu, senses and mind are purified."

Basti completely washes the bowel and removes excess bacteria, old stool, thread worms and heat from the lower intestines. Most importantly, it pushes apana vayu upward. When the apana, rises it can be felt in the navel and as a great pressure on the stomach. Basti cures digestive disorders and is particularly useful for removing constipation, controlling nervous diarrhoea and strengthening the solar plexus. It also improves muscle tone and blood supply as well as purifying the blood.

Basti should not be practised by anyone with high blood pressure, hernia or any serious digestive ailments. It is useful in treating ailments such as colitis and dysentery. However, in some cases it may be too drastic, so if you suffer from these types of disorders you should seek expert guidance.

Herbs and Substances used for Basti

The traditional Ayurvedic enema often utilizes an herbal decoction of Dashamul tea. This is a "10 root" formula that is a powerful pacifier for Vata dosha and all its related disorders. Although this tends to be the most commonly used formula, many herbs can be used, depending on the issues and imbalances at hand. In fact, the Dashamul can even be mixed with other herbs to form a more appropriate formula. For instance, if one is experiencing a Pitta imbalance, often the Dashamul tea can be blended with Guduchi, one of the main herbs for combating Pitta. Alternatively, one can mix Punarnava with the Dashamul during a Kapha imbalance. In general, most herbs can be administered through Basti, depending on the needs of the individual, their Prakruti (constitution) and their Vikruti (current imbalance).

The Ayurvedic enema is very a effective way of administering the herbs due to the direct absorption that takes place into the colon. At times however, other substances can be used as well. Other common medical substances include ghee, medicated ghee, or sesame oil. Using an oil base for the enema is called Anuvasan Basti, meaning with oil. Alternatively, the herbal decoction version is called Niruha Basti, meaning without oil. The oil method is most useful in disturbances that do not involve toxins (ama). If toxins are present, it is crucial to avoid the use of oil or ghee, as these substances can drive the toxins deeper into the tissues. If there are no signs of toxins, using oils or ghee can be a very powerful way to reduce Vata, anxiety, dryness, constipation and general depletion of the tissues. At times, these methods may be alternated in order to receive the benefits of both therapies.

Besides the herbal decoction or the oil enema, a few other medicinal substances that are used with the various Basti therapies include milk, medicated milk, bone broth, meat broth, herbal juices, honey (blended in the oil), egg whites, salt water, and even cow's urine. Each substance possesses specific health benefits and therefore, depending on the individual's needs, you can choose the medicine that would be most needed at any given time. In general, the traditional Dashamul Basti can be used for a wide range of body types and issues, making this a preferred "go-to" option by many.

Use of Basti

Basti can be used to treat just about any Vata disorder. In fact, it is just about the most powerful and effective way to treat Vata due to the direct application into the colon (aka the "home" of Vata). Common Vata disorders include anxiety, fear, restless mind, sleep disorders, nervous system disorders (i.e. Parkinson's), hypersensitivity, constipation, chronic gas and bloating, debility, depletion, emaciation, sciatica, gout, arthritis, osteoporosis, and dryness, to name a few. Further, since Vata is typically involved in other doshic imbalances as the primary movement force, the Basti can be used to indirectly alleviate both Pitta and Kapha, treating a wide variety of disorders and imbalances.

Another main indication to utilize the Basti therapy would be during times of cleansing. In fact, it is one of the main cleansing therapies of the traditional Pancha Karma (lit. the five cleansing actions) therapy. It is often used in many home cleanses such as the kitchari cleanse or a modified home "PK" (pancha karma) as well. Due to the direct application into the colon, the enema is quite effective in flushing out toxins from the intestines, making it a useful therapy for detoxification. When using the Basti for cleansing, one can use the traditional Dashamul decoction, or a blend of Dashamul with a cleansing herb such as Guduchi, Musta or Kutki. If there are thought to be parasites, it is highly recommended to use an anti-parasitical herb such as Vidanga for beneficial results.

When performing Basti during a cleanse, it is necessary to have gone through the typical "pre-cleanse" practices such as sweating (svedana) and oiliation (snehana).

Contraindications of Basti

Since the Basti is a relatively "invasive" therapy, one should use knowledge, awareness and precaution before performing. Here is a non-exhaustive list of some common contraindications for Basti:

- Pregnancy.
- Menstruation.
- Acute diarrhea.
- Hemorrhoids or rectal polyps.
- Within 2-3 hours after food intake.
- Shortness of breath.
- Rectal or vaginal prolapse.
- Ascites.
- Only a nutritive Basti should be done with severe debility or emaciation (i.e. bone marrow broth).

Frequency of Performing the Basti

How often one should perform the Basti will depend on a case by case basis. If you are treating a severe or chronic disorder, it is likely you will need to perform this multiple times over a prolonged period in order to receive the results you are needing. This can mean performing multiple days in a row consistently, or several days a week for a specific amount of weeks. It is important to avoid overdoing it with the Basti, as one can become habituated to the cleansing effect, weakening the colon overtime. Therefore it is usually best to give breaks in between, even with severe disorders.

During an Ayurvedic cleanse the Basti is typically performed 2-3 days consistently, and then once a week for about 4 weeks during the "post-cleanse" phase. After the cleanse, the Anuvasana (Oil) Basti can be used (if appropriate), as long as the toxins have been cleared out thoroughly.

If you are treating an acute or less severe disorder, one can perform the Basti 2-3 days consistently. If the imbalance still remains, wait 5-7 days and repeat until the disorder is removed.

Basti Instructions

1. Place the medicine of choice into the enema bag.
2. Hang the bag using a hanger or similar gadget up at a high elevation, ideally at least 6-9 feet up.
3. Lay a towel or an old sheet on the floor and have a pillow and blanket nearby to

keep comfortable after the application.

4. Have an empty container or jar at hand. Open the tube over the empty jar, letting the tea move down it, filling the entire tube completely before the insertion. This is a really quick open and close, so be prepared to close quickly to avoid wasting too much liquid. This step is important to let out any air in the tube, avoiding air coming into the colon.
5. Place a small amount of oil or ghee on the end of the tube to allow easy insertion.
6. Lay on your left side and insert the end of the enema tube into the rectum about 2 inches, keeping the tube closed.
7. Open the tube and allow the liquid to flow into the colon.
8. Once the bag is completely empty, close the tube, remove it from the rectum and place it in a safe place.
9. Lay on your left side for 5-10 minutes.
10. Switch to the right side for 5-10 minutes.
11. Place the pillow behind you and lay in a supported supine position. Stay here for as long as you feel comfortable.
12. The herbal enema may be retained indefinitely if the colon is really dry; this is totally fine. Otherwise, try to retain it for a minimum of 30 minutes or longer if possible. If there is too much pressure before then, just retain as long as possible to allow the absorption of the medicine into the colon.
13. To clean the bag, rinse out immediately after use with hot water in the tub. Once all of the sediment is removed, get out as much water as possible and then hang to dry.

Kapalabhati

'Kapala' is a Sanskrit word; it means skull. 'Bhati' means to shine. The term 'Kapalabhati' means an exercise that makes the skull shine. This Kriya cleanses the skull. So this is taken as one of the Shat-Karmas (six cleansing processes in Hatha Yoga).

Sit on Padmasana. Keep the hands on knees. Close the eyes. Perform Puraka and Rechaka rapidly. This should be practised vigorously. One will get perspiration profusely. This is a good form of exercise. Those who are well-versed in Kapalabhati can do Bhastrika very easily. There is no Kumbhaka in this Pranayama. Rechaka plays a prominent part. Puraka should be done quickly and forcibly by contracting the abdominal muscles with a backward push. When you do Puraka, release the abdominal muscles. Some people naturally make a curve of the spine and bend their heads also. This is not desirable. The head and the trunk should be erect. Sudden expulsions of breath follow one another as in Bhastrika. To start with, you can have one expulsion per second. Gradually you can have two expulsions per second. To begin with do one round in the morning consisting of 10 expulsions only. In the second week, do one round in the evening. In the third week, do two rounds in the morning and two rounds in the evening. Thus every week, gradually and cautiously increase 10 expulsions to each round till you get 120 expulsions for each round.

It cleanses the respiratory system and the nasal passages. It removes the spasm in bronchial tubes. Consequently, Asthma is relieved and also cured in course of time. The apices of the lungs get proper oxygenation. Thereby they cannot afford favourable nidus (breeding grounds) for tubercle bacilli. Consumption is cured by this practice. Lungs are considerably developed. Carbon dioxide is eliminated in a large scale. Impurities of the blood are thrown out. Tissues and cells absorb a large quantity of oxygen. The practitioner keeps up good health. Heart functions properly. The circulatory and respiratory systems are toned to a considerable degree.

Steps of Kapal Bhati Pranayama

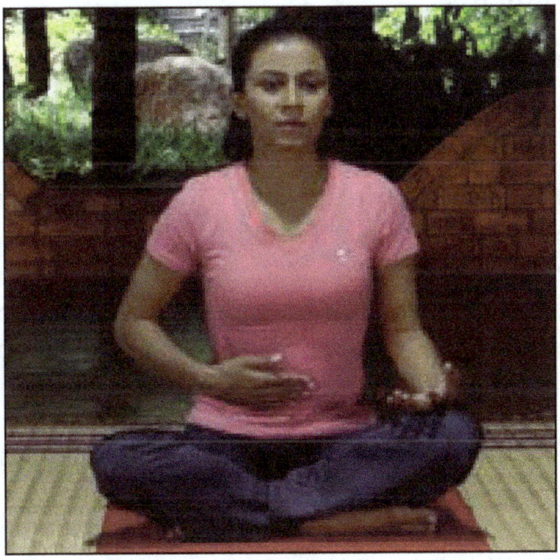

- Sit comfortably with your spine erect. Place your hands on the knees with palms open to the sky.
- Take a Deep Breath in.
- As you exhale, pull your stomach. Pull your navel in back towards the spine. Do as much as you comfortably can. You may keep your right hand on the stomach to feel the abdominal muscles contract.

- As you relax the navel and abdomen, the breath flows into your lungs automatically.
- Take 20 such breaths to complete one round of Kapal Bhati Pranayama.
- After completing the round, relax with your eyes closed and observe the sensations in your body.
- Do two more rounds of Kapal Bhati Pranayama.

Beginner's Kapalbhati Yoga Pranayama (Kapal Bhati Breathing Exercise)

To practice this breathing exercise sit up in a comfortable position, cross legged is best:

- Elongate your spine upwards, lengthen your neck and subtly bring your chin back and in like a soldier at attention. This will align the spine with the back of your head.
- Close your eyes.
- Have your hands in Gyan Mudra. In Gyan Mudra have your thumb tips and index finger meeting, with the wrists resting gently on the knees and the palms turned slightly upwards.
- Relax your stomach muscles.
- Now expel the air as forcefully as you are comfortable with through the nose. This should cause the abdominal muscles to contract sharply and should draw the abdomen inwards towards the spine (like when you suck in your stomach). Then allow the inhalation to occur completely passively without any additional effort. To repeat, the exhalation is done using conscious sharp force, while the inhalation is just a recoil action bringing the air back into the lungs. All the breathing takes place through the nose. Right after the passive inhalation, exhale again forcefully and continue at a steady rhythm.
- Do a round of 10 repetitions.
- Work your way up to doing 5 rounds, while taking a break between each round.
- Practice Note: Unlike doing Bhastrika Yoga Pranayama you use force during both the inhalation and the exhalation, in Kapalbhati force is only to be used during the exhalation.

Intermediate Kapalbhati Yoga Pranayama (Kapal Bhati Breathing Exercise)

Once you feel comfortable with the Beginner's version of Kapalbhati Yoga Pranayama, perform the breathing exercise with more force if possible and also increase the number of repetition per round to 50. You may also prefer to do a single round, but, with many more repetitions instead (up to 5 minutes worth).

Advanced Kapalbhati Yoga Pranayama (Kapal Bhati Breathing Exercise)

Build up to doing this pranayama for 15 minutes straight or equivalent number of rounds with more repetitions per rounds.

Secret of Kapalbhati Yoga Pranayama (Kapal Bhati Breathing Exercise)

The secret of the success of Kapalbhati Yoga Pranayama lies in where your mind is when doing this terrific breathing exercise. If you need to cure your body, then with every exhalation imagine that disease is being purged from your system. If you need to regain emotional balance, then again, with every exhalation visualize the negative emotions or weaknesses being thrown out of your system. If negative thoughts are the issue, let every exhalation expel them from your heart and mind.

Kapalbhati Pranayama Benefits for Health

Kapalbhati for Weight Loss - The Best Breathing Exercise

If you ask any yoga guru for the best breathing exercise in yoga for weight loss, without any hesitation they would say Kapalbhati. Yes, this is the best way to reduce weight fast. And this is completely natural.

Many studies has proved that people who did Kapalabhati daily had reduced their weight by more than 10 Kgs in less than 45 days. Even top Yoga gurus like Sri Baba Ramdev Ji, Bharat Thakur and many others recommend this as the best yoga technique for weight loss. Now don't be late. If you are one among those people suffering from obesity, try this breathing technique to reduce your body weight. You may also try other yoga poses like vajrasana, halasana along with this for better results. Be sure you follow a good veg diet too. And if you could stricly follow these, I am sure you can loss your weight by more than 10 to 15 Kgs in 45 days.

Cures Constipation

Though constipation sounds funny, it is one major problem for aged people. Their digestive fire is not so good and this leads to poor digestion. Constipation is not only a serious problem in old people, but also for kids and few young people.

Constipation leads to unhealthy lifestyle, various allergies, diarrhoea, swollen abdomen and many other health problems. Though there are some medicines to cure constipation, they are not good for longtime usage and they got many side effects too.

So for people who are facing constipation problem, Kapalbhati Pranayama is a best natural remedy. Do this for 3 to 5 minutes depending on your ability. And I promise you will be cured in less than 7 days. Also try dog breathing, vajrasana and sun salutations along this for better results.

Treats Breast Cancer

This may sound a little shocking. But it's true. According to a recent study, researchers had found that Kapalabhati Pranayama is effective in treating Breast Cancer.

Major reasons for Breast cancer are obesity, female sex, lack of any kind of exercises, alcohol consumption and many other. Breast Cancer is one major health problem among women in many western countries like United Sates, United Kingdom, Australia, Canada and in some other. They spend millions of dollars on Breast Cancer treatment.

But you know what, you can cure it naturally with the help of Kapalbhati. But remember that you should be in starting stage. if it is in final stage, you should go for some advanced laser treatments.

Improves Blood Circulation

Low blood circulation can cause many problems like skin allergies, cold hands, loss of hair, dry nails and many other. This may some times leads to serious health condition and you might need some advanced treatments.

But before it get worse, take some action. Kapalbhatti Pranayama is one good yoga technique to cure low blood circulation. It improves blood circulation for total body and keeps you healthy. So from today itself, start doing it for 3 to 5 minutes on either early mornings or evenings. Along this practice anulom vilom pranayam for faster benefits.

Strengthens Stomach Muscles

During Kapalbhati we forcefully exhale air from the body and during this process we forcefully push the stomach inside. As we keep pushing and relaxing, the muscles around abdomen gets exercised. And by this they get strengthened.

Natural Remedy for Nerves Weakness

Nerves weakness is another common problem seen in many people today. Due to improper intake of food, over stress, less sleep and unhealthy lifestyle, people of almost all ages face this problem. This further leads to fatigue, low energy levels, headaches, impotency, infertility and many other problems.

And according to many yoga gurus, Kapalabhati pranayam is a perfect breathing exercise for curing nerves weakness problem. With this pranayam almost all nerves in your body gets energised and gets stable. And according to reports, practising Kapalbhati pranayam for 25 to 30 days continuously can treat nerves weakness completely.

Increases Immunity Power

The main reason for people getting attacked to various diseases like fever, sinus, cough and other easily is low immunity power. The more immunity power you have, the more you stay healthy. Whatever the capsules or tonics you use while attacked to these diseases is to increase your immnity power.

And what if you can increase your immunity power yourself at home with free of cost. It will be amazing right. For this what all you need to do is to practice Kapalbhati pranayam 3 to 4 rounds everyday.

Increases Sex Stamina and Sperm Count

Kapalbhati pranayam is also know for increasing sex moods and sperm count. Many yoga gurus suggest this for infertility and other sex problems. Practising this pranayam daily makes the body parts around abdomen fit and helps performing well during sexual intercourse. This even calms your mind and increases you moods and libido.

Cures Lungs Problems

In this highly polluted era, 10 out of every 100 people suffer from various kinds of lungs problems. Reasons could be many like smoking, alcohol consumption, dust pollution, body fat - but one should be alert. Weak lungs can be a risk for your life.

So if you are one among those suffering from weak lungs and other lungs problems, practice Kapalabhati for 3 to 5 minutes daily both and early mornings and evenings. All your lungs problems can be cured in less than 20 days. But be sure to take advice from your doctor. It is not recommended for people suffering from serious lung patients because it is difficult for them. You can also do anulom vilom along this for better results.

Treats Periods Problems in Women

Kapalbhati Pranayama is really a gift to women. This simple breathing yoga exercise works like magic for many diseases commonly seen in women. Many women suffer from improper periods problem. Sometimes they occur very fast and some other times slow. For this they run after various medications and drugs.

But you know what, practising this Pranayama for 10 to 15 days continuously can cure this problem naturally without any cost. Yes, this is tried by thousands of women and worked successfully for most of them. Even Swami Baba Ramdev has mentioned this in one of his Hindi speech video. So now its your turn to give a try.

Cures Kidney Stones Problems

Stones in Kidneys has joined into one other common diseases these days. Taking from old people to young people, it is affecting everyone. Though there is cure for this problems, big hospitals charge a lot for this.

But Kapalbhati Pranayama can cure stones in kidneys without any cost. This is a proven yoga technique for kidney stones. Yoga master like Swami Baba Ramdev had treated a lot of people with this problem. Of course, you also need to follow some good ayurvedic diet to treat it completely.

For Bone Strength

Low levels of calcium in body can lead to bone weakness. And we commonly see this bone problems in aged people and women. For this doctors suggest some calcium tablets and other calcium rich foods. Besides consuming these, practising Kapalbhati can also increasing calcium levels in your body and make your bones strong.

This not only makes your bones strong, but it even helps in fighting other bone related diseases too. Just try this for 2 weeks and you will be amazed with the results.

Treats Uterine Fibroids in Women

Uterine Fibroids is a commonly seen problem in women. Fibroids gets developed in the muscular wall of uterus and this leads to increase in uterus size, heavy bleeding, pain while having sex and some other problems. For this doctors suggest some kid of western medicines and in some cases they go for surgery.

But Baba Ramdev had proved that they could be cured by Kapalabhati Pranayama. He himself mentioned this in his Kapalbhati hindi speech. But the patient should do more rounds. It should be practised for 15 minutes (900 exhales) continuously without any break. The more dangerous the disease is the more exhales you need.

Cures Acidity Problems

Bad food habits and improper food timings can lead to acidity problems and put you in trouble. And this leads to indigestion, heart burn, stomach burn and other throat, stomach problems. Even for this you don't need to run after doctors and medicines. Just do Kapalabhati for 5 minutes daily and all your acidity problems will be cleared away in less than 2 weeks.

Increases Energy Levels

If you are one among those people with low energy levels, then you need this breathing exercise. These days people get tired and weak soon. They run after many energy drinks like Red Bull, Monster, KS and many other for energy. But they are unaware that this simple yoga breathing technique can increase their energy levels by 3 times than that of those artificial energy drinks.

Benefits of Kapalbhati for Skin and Beauty

Best Breathing Exercise for Natural Skin Glow

If you are searching for any best breathing techniques of yoga for naturally glowing skin ? Then I recommend Kapalabhati for that. Not only me, even great yoga gurus and beauty experts suggest this for white and bright skin.

At first, I was a little confusing on this. But I personally tried it for 20 days and got surprised with the results. And now I am addicted to it. Now I do it everyday for 5 to 10 minutes on evenings. Kapalbhati itself mean that glow on forehead (skull). So why late, just try this simple breathing technique from today and make your skin glow like never before in less than 3 weeks. Try anulom vilom along this for much better results.

Best Natural Yoga Technique to Cure Pimples

Wow, super amazing right ? So, Kapalbhati can even cure pimples. Pimples are night mares for many young boys and girls. And they spend most of their time on searching for some best ways to cure them. Now you don't need to search for any beauty products to cure pimple. You can cure them yourself at your home without spending a single dollar on it.

Yes, what all you need to do is to do Kapalbhatti for 5 to 7 minutes depending on your energy and time. While doing this, you exhale forcefully and by this a huge amount of blood is pumped to face. This clears all the impure blood in face part and cures pimples. And I am sure all your pimple problems will be cured in less than 10 days with this simple technique.

Treats Vascular Veins on Face

Vascular veins on face can make you look ugly and spoil your beautiful face. One of the reasons for Vascular veins is poor blood circulation to head part. And with Kapalbhatti Pranayama you pump huge amount of blood to skull and by this all the vascular veins will be cleared in less than 30 days.

Slows Ageing

Almost all Pranayama yoga techniques are capable of slowing ageing process. And among them, Kapalbhati can be known as king. Anti ageing is one of the best kapalbhati benefits.

People who practice this yoga breathing exercise look 8 to 10 years younger than their age. This is scientifically proven yoga technique.

Benefits of Kapalbhati for Hair

Prevents Hair Loss

Wow, it can prevent hair loss too. You might be a little surprised with this benefit of Kapalbhatti, but its 100% true. This yoga pranayama technique increases blood flow to skull (head part) and makes the roots of hair strong. If the roots of hair are strong, you will never experience hair loss. So if you are aiming for strong and long hair, practice this breathing exercise daily for few minutes. Along this practise Balayam Yoga technique for 5 to 10 minutes daily for better results.

Prevents Premature Hair Greying

If you could observe closely, these days almost all men and women suffer from premature hair greying problem. Our hair is losing its original color and turns grey or white at the early ages of 20 and 22. Even for this problem, Kapalabhati works well. Along this you can also try Balayam (nail rubbing yoga technique for better results).

Kapalbhati Benefits for Mind

Calms Mind

Overthinking can lead to mental stress and cause a lot of problems. For this breathing exercises are best natural remedy. And among all breathing techniques, Kapalbhati works well for this. So just practice it for 5 to 10 minutes and experience the peace and bliss hidden in you.

To Treat Stress and Anxiety

Increased work pressure, mental tensions and other bad lifestyles could lead to mind related diseases like stress and anxiety. This is completely common and you don't need any drugs for these. What all I suggest is to do Kapalabhati daily.

Cures Insomnia

Though there might be a lot of reasons for insomnia (sleepless ness), most of them are related to mind. If you are mind is calm and perfect, then you could sleep well. If it keep on disturbing you, then you can't sleep. So for this problem, practise Kapalabhati for 5 to 8 minutes on evenings. It can seriously cure insomnia.

Kundalini Jagaran

Last but not the least, for Kundalini awakening. Though pranayam has many health and beauty benefits, the primary reason why yogis do pranayama is for Kundalini awakening. And with Kapalbhati you can awaken the Kundalini energy from Muladhara chakra to Sahasrara chakra. And with this you can get enormous powers and reach samadhi. This stands top among the kapalbhati benefits.

People who Should Avoid doing Kapal Bhati Pranayama

Avoid practicing this breathing technique if you have an artificial pacemaker or stent, epilepsy, hernia, backache due to slip disc, or have recently undergone abdominal surgery.

Women should not practice Skull Shining Breathing technique during and shortly after pregnancy as well as during menstruation as it involves vigorous abdominal squeezes.

People with hypertension and heart problems should practice this breathing technique only under a yoga expert's guidance.

Cautions

Kapalabhati Pranayama is an advanced breathing technique. Do not attempt it if you are not proficient with basic pranayamas, such as Three-Part Breath (Dirga Pranayama) and Ocean Breath (Ujjayi Pranayama). Also avoid practicing Kapalabhati if you currently have high blood pressure, heart disease, or a hernia. Women who are pregnant should avoid practicing this exercise, as well. As with all breathing exercises, always approach the practice with caution, especially if you have a respiratory condition, such as asthma or emphysema.

Never attempt any pranayama for the first time without the guidance of a qualified and knowledgeable teacher. Stop the exercise if you become faint or dizzy. Always work within your own range of limits and abilities. If you have any medical concerns, talk with your doctor before practicing yoga.

Trataka

Trataka is a Hatha Yoga method to develop concentration. Trataka is a simple, yet powerful practice and is one of the six purification methods or Shatkarmas, taught in Hatha Yoga. The technique has to do with gazing or fixing the eyes on one point, either on an object or on a candle flame.

The practice of Trataka is based on the scientific fact, that the movement of the eyeballs can reflect our thinking process. When we concentrate, our thoughts are focused on a particular subject due to which, the stray thoughts become less or may even vanish. At the same time the eyeballs become steadier. There is a connection between our eyeball movement and our mental state. This can be easily demonstrated on an EEG machine.

The same principle is used in the practice of Trataka. If we forcefully fix our gaze on a particular point, we can induce a steady concentrated mind. Our thoughts will become less and the turbulent mind can be brought under control.

There are many types of Trataka. Practitioners use many different objects for doing steady gazing. Flame of a candle, a black dot on the wall, the crystal ball, the Shiva Linga, the early morning sun, the full moon, picture of a deity, etc. can be used depending on one's choice. The most commonly followed technique is gazing on a candle flame.

This can be done in two ways:

1. Bahya Trataka.
2. Antar Trataka.

Bahya Trataka

The eyes are kept open and concentrate on some objects like rising or setting sun, moon and stars. Selection of object has to be based on expert guidance.

Antar Trataka

Here the eyes are closed and concentration should be directed to the Chakras of our body viz. the navel, the region of the heart, the centre of the brows.

Preparation

- Get candle, candle stand and matchbox.
- Wash your eyes with cool and clean water (with eye cup if available) before starting the practice for good result.
- When you practice in a group, sit around the candle stand, making a circle at adequate distance from the candle stand (1.5 to 2 mts.) The maximum number of participants in a group around could be ten. Keep the candle at the same level as the eyes.

Instructions

- Sit in any comfortable meditative posture, if required you may sit in a chair.
- Remove your glasses and wrist watch.
- Keep your spine, neck and head erect in a line. Collapse your shoulders.
- Close your eyes and adopt Namaskara mudra (join both the palms and place them on the chest with the thumb touching the sternum).
- Keep smiling throughout the practice. Calm down your mind. Observe your body and breath.

Preparatory Eye Exercises

Up and Down or Vertical Movements

- Open your eyes with a few blinks.
- Gently move your eyeballs up-down. Do it ten times. Move your eyeballs smoothly and continuously. Try to avoid jerky movements and keep your head steady. Practise at your own pace.

Right and Left or Horizontal Movement of Eyeballs

- Gently open your eyes with a few blinks.
- Gently move your eyeballs right- left. Do it ten times. Move your eyeballs smoothly and continuously. Try to avoid jerky movements and keep your head steady. Practise at your own pace.
- After completing ten rounds gently stop the practice and close your eyes.
- Rub your palms against each other, form a cup of your palms and cover your eyes.
- Practise simple palming. Do not touch the eyelids with your palms directly . Relax your eye muscles completely. Relax for a while.
- Feel the warmth and darkness in your eyes. Ensure that your eyes are totally in dark.
- After sufficient relaxation, gently drop your hands down.
- Feel the cool sensation around the eyeballs. Relax for a while. Do not open your eyes immediately.

Diagonal Movement of Eyeballs

- Open your eyes with a few blinks.
- Gently move your eyeballs to extreme right up, extreme left down. Do it ten times. Move your eyeballs smoothly and continuously. Try to avoid jerky movements and keep your head steady. Practise at your own pace.
- After completing ten rounds gently stop the practice and close your eyes.
- Rub your palms against each other, form a cup of your palms and cover your eyes.
- Give press and release palming.

- After completing five rounds, gently drop your hands down.
- Feel the cool sensation around the eyeballs. Relax for a few seconds. Do not open your eyes immediately.
- Rotational movement of the eyeballs.

Clockwise Movement

- Open your Eyes with A Few Blinks.
- Gently move your eyeballs to the left, up, right, down; Left-up, right-down. Do it ten times. Move your eyeballs smoothly and continuously. Try to avoid jerky movements and keep your head steady. Practise at your own pace.
- After completing ten rounds gently stop the practice and close your eyes.
- Rub your palms against each other, form a cup of your palms and cover your eyes.
- Give constant pressure palming. Press constantly around the eyeballs with your palms. Inhale deeply and exhale completely. Do not press on the eyeballs. Relax your eye muscles completely.
- After completing five rounds of deep slow breathing, gently drop your hands down.
- Feel the cool sensation around the eyeballs. Relax for a few seconds. Do not open your eyes immediately.

Anti Clockwise Movement

- Now, proceed to anti-clockwise rotation of the eyeballs.
- Open your eyes with a few blinks.
- Gently move your eyeballs in anti clockwise direction right, up, left, down; right-up, left-down. Do it ten times. Move your eyeballs smoothly and continuously. Try to avoid jerky movements and keep your head steady. Practise at your own pace.
- After completing ten rounds gently stop the practice and close your eyes.
- Rub your palms against each other, form a cup of your palms and cover your eyes.
- Give constant pressure palming.

- If you feel like changing your position, you may do so. Take rest for sometime before you start Jyoti Trataka.

Jyoti Trataka

Step 1 Effortless Gazing or Focusing at Flame

- Gently open your eyes with a few blinks and look at the floor. Do not look at the flame directly.
- Slowly shift your vision to the base of the candle stand, then move to the top of the stand, then to the candle and then slowly look at the flame of the candle. Now, start gazing at the whole flame without any effort. Do not blink your eyes. There may be some irritating sensation, but use your will power and gaze in a relaxed way. If tears appear, allow it to flow freely. This is a sign of good practice. Let the tears wash out the impurities from the eyes. Learn to ignore the irritation and watering from the eyes.
- Gaze at the flame for about 30 seconds.
- Slowly close your eyes, rub your palms against each other for a few seconds, form a cup of your palms and cover your eyeballs.
- Give press and release palming.
- After completing five rounds, gently drop your hands down.
- Feel the cool sensation around the eyeballs. Relax for a while. Do not open your eyes immediately.

Step 2 Intensive Focusing at the Tip of the Wick of the Flame

- Gently open your eyes with a few blinks and look at the floor. Do not look at the flame directly.
- Slowly shift your vision to the base of the candle stand, then move to the top of the stand, then to the candle and then slowly look at the flame of the candle. Now, start gazing at the whole flame without any effort.
- Slowly gaze at the tip of the wick of the candle. Focus your attention at one point. This is a practice of focusing and concentration. Keep on gazing, use your will power. Let the tears come out and try not to blink your eyes. By practice the gaze becomes steady, making the mind one pointed.
- Gaze at the flame for about 30 seconds.
- Slowly close your eyes, rub your palms against each other for a few seconds then form a cup of your palms and cover your eyes.

- Give constant pressure palming. Press constantly around the eyeballs with your palms and inhale deeply and exhale completely. Continue four more rounds. Do not touch the eyeballs with your palms directly. Relax your eye muscles completely.
- After completing five rounds, gently drop your hands down.
- Feel the cool sensation around the eyeballs. Relax for a few seconds. Do not open your eyes immediately.
- Continuously gaze at the flame, no blinking or winking, smooth and effortless gazing.
- Use your will power and ignore watering or irritation in the eyes. Gradually increase the duration of gazing upto 60 seconds over a few weeks of practice.

Step 3 De-focusing

- Gently open your eyes with a few blinks and look at the floor. do not look at the flame directly.
- Slowly shift your vision to the base of the candle stand then move to the top of the stand, then to the candle and then slowly look at the flame of the candle. First fix your attention at the flame, then gradually widen your vision. Slowly de focus your attention from the flame and have a defocused gaze on the flame. With expansive awareness, collect all the details of the flame such as the colour of the flame, shape of the flame and aura around the flame. Then observe the aura expanding more and more and see the small light particles around the flame.
- After one minute of de-focusing, gaze or focus on the flame. Slowly close your eyes and retain the image in your mind. Visualize the flame between your eyebrows and collect all the details with your eyes closed. When the image disappear go for palming.
- This time palming is combines with breathing and Bhramari.
- First apply constant pressure around the eyes, then inhale and chant Bhramari Mmmmm, feel the vibrations of Bhramari throughout the body; repeat the same. Inhale-chant Mmmmmmm, as you exhale. Feel the sound resonance in the entire head region especially around the eye region.

Step 4 Silence

- Feel the silence and relax for a while. After sufficient relaxation, gently drop your hands down. Sit quiet for some time and feel the deep comforting effect of the practice. Be aware of the changes taking place inside you. Recognize that the mind has become completely calm, your concentration, will power and sharpness of eyesight has improved.

- Gently bring your hands behind the back, catch hold of the right wrist with your left palm, make a loose fist with the right hand and feel the pulse of the right hand.
- As you breathe out, gently bend down towards the floor and surrender to the All mighty.
- Come back as you breathe in.
- Gently give a feather massage around the eye muscles with three fingers (index, middle and ring fingers).

Tips for Practitioners

- This practice is to be done in the dark preferably in the evening.
- Remove glasses, wristwatch and belt and make yourself comfortable in the posture.
- Sit with your head, neck and spine erect. always open your eyes with a few blinks.
- During eye exercises head is not to be moved but the eyeballs.
- During Jyoti Trataka, when you open the eyes, don't look at the flame right away. Start looking at the floor and then slowly bring your gaze onto the flame.
- During palming don't let the palms touch or press the eyeballs (Palms and not the fingers cover the eyes).
- Breathe slowly and deeply with awareness during palming.
- Palms are placed in such a way that there is complete darkness in front of eyes.
- The facial muscles, eyebrows and eyelids should remain totally relaxed.
- Trataka should be performed after Asanas and Pranayama.
- Practise Trataka on a steady flame.
- Avoid undue strain to the eyes.

Benefits of Trataka

The trataka exercises including the nosetip gaze, eyebrow centre gaze and right and left shoulder gaze, etc., especially train and strengthen the eye muscles- particularly the four pairs of muscles controlling the upward, downward, right and left movements of the eyeballs. Defects of vision and other eye troubles, which force people to use glasses or contact lenses, are cured by trataka. Gazing at various objects of nature accustoms the eyes to the varied influences of light and environments etc. The eye muscles generally act asymmetrically in the ordinary use of the eyes, and thus produce eye strain or weariness, which further aggravates visionary troubles. The regular and systematic practice of various eye exercises of trataka can correct all these. Trataka can increase the vision so much so that even the smallest particle in the dead darkness (and also in the dazzling light) becomes visible. Inflammation of the eyes, trachoma, styes, astigmatism, myopia, hypermetropia and presbyopia etc., in short all the eye problems can be corrected by trataka. Trataka vitalises vision by accelerating blood circulation in and around the area of the eyes, and also naturalises eye infections by destroying the microbes through tears.

By directing the gaze at the eyebrow centre, the olfactory nerves and the optic nerves are stimulated, and as a result, the autonomic and the central nervous systems are awakened. There is a close relationship between mind and vision, thus trataka not only maintains the physical health of eyes but also helps a great deal in controlling the mind. It causes a soothing effect on the cranial nerves, thus enabling the mind to become one-pointed. It greatly improves memory and willpower, and helps to attain perfection in samyama (i.e. dharana, dhyana, samadhi) described in Patanjala Yoga. Laboratory tests on trataka have proved that it brings back certain repressed experiences to the level of consciousness. For ocular health, in addition to the trataka practice, stroking, moving, pressing, palming, light kneading and salakyam (as described in Satkarma-sangrahah) of the eyes are also quite beneficial.

Precautions

1. Trataka, like other intricate yogic exercises should be learned under the direct guidance of some accomplished yoga guru; otherwise there is every possiblity that eye muscles as well as the nervous system may be damaged.

2. Eyes should be splashed and washed with cold water immediately after the trataka practice. This will stimulate the blood supply in the eye regions.

3. Avoid using external eye medicine or solution after trataka. Also avoid rubbing the eyes, even if in the beginning of trataka you feel some eye strain, which would be due to adaptation to eye exercises.

4. Avoid doing trataka on the burning sun. For better eye health, it is advised to sit with closed eyes, facing the sun. Trataka on the sun with open eyes should be performed in the early morning and late afternoon (i.e. sunset). However, trataka on the full moon of puma-mashi is the best.

5. Some bodily exercises before and after trataka are necessary to revitalise the tissues and nerves.

6. The continuous repetition and reflection upon the symbol of Isvara i.e. Aum, during trataka practice will be very beneficial spiritually.

Trataka Contraindications

The practice of Trataka (Candle Gazing) is more towards a meditative practice, and no doubt the benefits are derived from deep long and repeated practices. But for beginners this practice needs to be done with care and with guidance from a yoga teacher (guru). Some of the main precautions are mentioned below:

- Migraine: As this practice involves constant staring without blinking, students who are new to this may overdo it. This when done by migraine patients will aggregate the irritation.
- Lack of control over the senses: Those who have issues in controlling their senses, may have problems when Trataka (Candle Gazing) is done. Working on improving the various sense organs with the activation of the nerves through yoga poses practice becomes essential before the Trataka (Candle Gazing) practice.
- Trauma sensitive related issues: Patients suffering from trauma should be introduced to Trataka (Candle Gazing) gradually, as this could cause fear of staring, fear of the dark (while closing eyes), lack of self control, irritation with eyes watering etc.
- Surgery: Any kind of surgery related to the eyes should be avoided as this practice will cause pressure to the eye muscles.

References

- Sutra-neti-nasal-cleaning-in-hatha-yoga: yogicwayoflife.com, Retrieved 19,July 2020
- Top-Kapalbhati-Pranayam-Benefits: tipsmonk.com, Retrieved 31,March 2020
- Jala-neti-cleaning-your-sinuses: yogicwayoflife.com, Retrieved 29,May 2020
- kapalbhati-yoga-breathing-exercise-for-optimum-health-healing-free-online-pranayama-book-ch-5: anmolmehta.com, Retrieved 30,June 2020
- Basti-ayurvedic-enema-multitude-health-benefits-uses: svasthaayurveda.com, Retrieved 21,June 2020
- Nauli-kriya-abdominal-massage-in-hatha-yoga-shatkarma: yogicwayoflife.com, Retrieved 11,July 2020
- The-benefits-of-jala-neti: stevenaitchison.co.uk, Retrieved 09,May 2020

7

Yoga in Religion

In addition to being a set of physical and mental practices, yoga also comprises religious practices. It is an integral aspect of various religions in the Indian subcontinent such as Hinduism, Jainism and Buddhism. This chapter closely examines the relationship of yoga with these religions as well as its depiction in popular culture in order to provide an extensive understanding of the subject.

Yoga and Hinduism

Everyone accepts that Hinduism is permeated with yogic teachings, and so I will not spend too much time on this aspect of Yoga's heritage. What is important to realize, though, is that the word yoga did not acquire its well-known technical sense until about 1000 B.C. when it appeared in the Taittiriya Upanishad. From the context it is clear that it stood for the control of the senses and the mind. Prior to that, the term yoga was widely used in its many nontechnical meanings—"union," "conjunction," "team," "sum," "equipment," and so on.

Does this mean, then, that spiritual teachings did not exist in earlier times? Of course not. Already the Rig Veda, the oldest literary collection in the world, is bristling with spiritual ideas and practices which are an archaic form of Yoga. The ancient sages used the word tapas for these teachings, which means literally "heat" or "glow." It refers to all those many practices—along with their underlying ideas—by which the Vedic seers (rishis) sought to find immortality in the divine realm. As one seer expressed it to the God Indra: By performing austerities we win heaven itself.

Early Western scholars regarded the 10,440 verses of the Rig Veda as "primitive Nature poetry" from the childhood of humanity, with little significance or appeal. It was a modern-day sage, the Bengali philosopher-yogin. Sri Aurobindo, who aimed to correct this opinion by focusing on the spiritual content and great relevance of the Vedic hymns to human psychology. Gradually, a new perspective is emerging among Western academics. In Vedicist Jeanine Miller's words: "Vedic thought, especially with regard to meditation and eschatology, reveals an unexampled depth of insight into the intricacies of the human mind, the background philosophy of which was the root of all subsequent speculations."

The later, post-Vedic teachings of Yoga can be understood as directly evolving out of the earlier Vedic tradition of tapas. Many of the Rig Vedic beliefs and practices are recognizably present in subsequent teachings, if often in modified form. Even in post-Vedic times, the word tapas was occasionally used in place of yoga. This was also the case in Jainism and Buddhism, which formed in counterpoint to the Vedic stream of wisdom already within the Indian civilization.

Transcendental Meditation

On January 29, 1959, Maharishi Mahesh Yogi arrived at San Francisco International Airport. It was his first visit to the United States, and the second continent on his global tour to introduce his Transcendental Meditation technique to the world.

Maharishi lectured to hundreds of people during his 2-month stay; many people learned the technique. The San Francisco Chronicle covered one of Maharishi's lectures and published the first article on Transcendental Meditation ever in America. Maharishi's message then was simple and direct, and it's the same today. Life is bliss. Man is born to enjoy. Within everyone is an unlimited reservoir of energy, intelligence, and happiness. Transcendental Meditation is a simple, effortless procedure to experience it. The technique can be easily learned by anyone of any age, culture, religion, or educational background.

In those early days, there were no other Transcendental Meditation teachers, no Transcendental Meditation centers. After San Francisco, Maharishi spent several months in Los Angeles, then traveled on to New York. From New York, Maharishi went to England, Germany, Greece, and on around the world.

The Transcendental Meditation movement started simply and grew steadily. Then suddenly, with the first published scientific research on the technique, Transcendental Meditation gained worldwide recognition. The first study on Transcendental Meditation was conducted at the University of California at Los Angeles in 1968 by physiologist Robert Keith Wallace. His thesis, "The Physiological Effects of Transcendental Meditation: A Proposed Fourth Major State of Consciousness," earned him his Ph.D., and his findings were published in the journals Science and Scientific American. This also inspired a huge upsurge of research into the effects of Transcendental Meditation. By 1975 Transcendental Meditation was a household word. And today? More than four million people worldwide -- including more than one million people in the United States -- from every profession, age, educational background, and religion practice Transcendental Meditation. And the number keeps growing.

The technique has been learned by over 6,000 medical doctors in the U.S. and by tens of thousands of executives, managers, and employees of large corporations and small businesses throughout the U.S. and the world. Homemakers practice Transcendental Meditation. So do attorneys, computer programmers, teachers, students, sales clerks, clergy, athletes, factory workers, architects, airline pilots, electricians, chefs, and artists. During the past 25 years, more than 500 scientific research studies have been conducted on the effects of the Transcendental Meditation technique at 210 independent universities and research institutions in 33 countries. The studies - many of which have been published in leading scientific journals - have shown that the Transcendental Meditation program:

- Reduces stress.
- Increases creativity and intelligence.
- Improves memory and learning ability.
- Increases energy.
- Increases inner calm.
- Reduces insomnia.
- Increases happiness and self-esteem.
- Reduces anxiety and depression.
- Improves relationships.
- Improves health.
- Promotes a younger biological age.

Transcendental Meditation is not new, but is a part of the Vedic tradition of India, stretching back several thousand years. It is the heart of the Yoga system, and an important part of Ayurveda (the 'Science of Life'), the world's most ancient system of natural healthcare and personal development. It may not always have had the same name, but the same basic technique has appeared many times in the past. At times when it disappeared from popular awareness, it was always preserved by the monks of the Shankaracharya tradition as Raja Yoga, the 'royal path to unity', which described the vast mental resources that lie virtually untapped below the surface of our conscious mind.

Through misunderstanding of the origins of Transcendental Meditation original teachings however, the process prescribed to release this potential and thereby solve life's problems, Ashtanga Yoga, of which TM is described as the 'heart', has been interpreted as eight steps of control and correct behaviour, which would eventually lead to the ability to experience a settled mind or samadhi. Because of this confusion of cause and effect, it didn't work for all but a few who were prepared to give up normal activity. Meditation was for a long time relegated to the fringes of everyday life, and for active people became substituted by visualisation and other relaxation techniques.

In the 1950s, however, a major revival of interest in meditation began when Maharishi Mahesh Yogi, a disciple of a renowned leader of the Shankaracharya tradition, Swami

Brahmananda Saraswati, travelled throughout India and around the world several times to re-establish the original understanding of meditation as a simple, effortless flow of the mind towards happiness.

People's experience of the mind's natural tendency to be active had been leading them into efforts to control it, forgetting that it is also the nature of the mind to be still when given the opportunity. In order to distinguish his revival of the pure knowledge from the prevailing misunderstandings, he called it Transcendental Meditation (TM). More than six million people have discovered on learning TM, that the most advanced meditation (meaning the most effective) is actually the simplest and can be practised by anybody. So no effort is needed. In fact, the only rule given to new meditators is 'don't make an effort.' Quite a relief for most people.

Transcendental Meditation

Mantras

TM is practised by silently and effortlessly thinking a mantra or sound, which has been passed on during personal instruction by a fully-trained teacher following careful guidelines laid down by Maharishi Mahesh Yogi. It is strongly recommended that you do not try to learn TM from any other source, even if they claim to be using Transcendental Meditation mantras, for reasons which will become apparent below.

How do Transcendental Meditation Mantras Work?

The mantra does not act as a focus for the mind as in other forms of meditation, but as a 'vehicle' upon which the attention gently and innocently rests. This allows the mind to settle into increasingly subtle levels of thinking, and finally the mantra itself is transcended and we settle into silence.

There are two qualities of the Transcendental Meditation mantra which are important for this process to occur:

- It is a meaningless sound. Using a word with meaning would keep the mind on the surface, thinking about the word, and not allow it to transcend (go beyond) that level.
- Its vibration has a resonance with its source in the primordial hum (Om) close to the silent, blissful level of the mind which gives it a tendency to fade in that direction. This attracts and charms the mind, which itself is always searching for greater happiness, so the mind settles with the mantra towards silence.

Where do Transcendental Meditation Mantras Come from?

The mantras used in Transcendental Meditation come from the ancient Vedic tradition of India. They are Sanskrit sounds, the language which is the closest possible human imitation of the natural vibrations produced by the dynamism of the unified field – the field identified by objective modern science as the silent source of all creation, and by yogis in their meditation as the Self – the field of Pure Consciousness. Some mantras have healing power for specific parts of the body, but the Transcendental Meditation mantras are for transcending, which has an enormous healing effect for the whole body and mind and much more.

How do you Choose the Transcendental Meditation Mantra?

There are thousands of mantras, from which a small number with known effects are used. We choose one that is suitable for you from a selection passed on by Maharishi according to a simple procedure that ensures it is correct.

It is important to receive the mantra from a fully trained Transcendental Meditation teacher because they have been given a selection of mantras which have been passed down through a long line of teachers over thousands of years. The effects are therefore well known both historically and currently to be always positive and life-enhancing. The mantras and procedures for passing them on are received by the teacher after months of intensive training, and the student is asked not to share the mantra or the way it is taught with anyone. This is for the benefit of the one already meditating (see next question), and to preserve the purity of the teaching ensuring that every person receives full and correct instruction. This is very important.

There are 4 vital aspects of the teaching that ensure that it will work for you:

- Receiving a correct mantra.
- Knowing how to use it properly.
- Being able to correctly interpret the experiences that come as a result.
- Having the support and guidance of a fully trained teacher free for the rest of your life.

Any one of these aspects missing could result in incorrect practice, lack of progress, and giving up on meditation completely, so missing a priceless opportunity to significantly enhance your life.

This is not an uncommon feeling for people to have before they start. However after a few TM meditations, the mantra becomes very personal to you; it's the vehicle that allows the attention to dive inwards and the mind begins to associate the mantra with the experience of settling down and enjoying inner silence. It becomes a treasured and trusted friend. Speaking the mantra aloud, chanting it or passing it on is to bring the mantra 'out', to reverse its natural direction – it's of no value. Also, the Transcendental Meditation mantras only work in context. Using or speaking the mantra without its simple yet very specific instructions and personal guidance from a teacher simply doesn't work. Because the way that TM is taught is simple and does work, once you learn you will no doubt feel, as others have, that you want friends and family to learn it in the same simple, effective and enjoyable way. We find therefore that it is actually extremely rare for anyone to abuse their mantra in this way, even if they started with the same doubt as you.

Why Not Om?

As explained above, not just any sound will do. Different mantras have different effects. The mantras used in TM are a group of 'householder' mantras designed to enable people to experience deep, restful meditation which brings integration between inner silence and outer activity – deep rest along with energy and dynamism. Om has a strong environmental effect which is OK if chanted in a group, but if used as a personal, internal mantra, it is suited only for those wanting to withdraw from active life.

Isn't it Better to Chant the Mantra?

Chanting the mantra will keep the body (mouth, throat etc.) active, and therefore not allow it to sink into the state of natural, deep rest that TM is famous for. Chanting also controls the mind and prevents it from settling into silence, as it naturally wants to do. And modern science has shown us that these quieter, deeper levels of life are more powerful – the nuclear level is far more powerful than the atomic level. Similarly, mantras are more powerful when they are thought rather than chanted, but the biggest power is discovered when the mantra is transcended as in the process of Transcendental Medita.

How can we be Sure the Mantras Work?

You cannot get a wrong mantra if taught by a qualified TM teacher, and it will always work because it is a natural process. Extremely rarely someone feels the mantra is not right, but this is always a sign of incorrect use – and easily corrected by their teacher. These particular Transcendental Meditation mantras have been passed on in this specific way to millions of people all around the world since Maharishi's revival of this ancient knowledge in 1958. The success of the technique has been verified by the benefits indicated by testimonials and a vast body of scientific research in universities around the world.

How to do Transcendental Meditation?

Pure Mind Reflection for Self-Realization

Pure Mind Reflection is using the tool of reflection to dive deep within one's own small self or physical self, until the small self leaves this 3rd, 4th, and 5th dimension; for the 6th dimension. This is where the small self/physical self, hands itself off to the True Self or Soul. This is what is called "Dying to the World, Beatific Vision, Samadhi, Being Born Again, or being blessed by God with Self-Realization" -- the knowledge of God the Absolute, the Father, Holy Spirit, and the Son.

As the mind begins it is impure. By that I mean it is completely full of all types of thoughts. As one moves through the meditation process, the mind purifies itself. By that I mean it begins to have less and less thoughts, which interrupt concentration. Thoughts are the mind's wants, which are caused by desires the five senses create within us all. As you meditate day after day, the mind begins to want less and less. This is the mind beginning to not want this world. Doing this over time will take you beyond time and space.

When the mind is finally pure, it is done wanting the physical world. These only needs to happen for one single instant and you will have transported yourself into the pure mind of the 6th dimension. Where, out of God comes a witness, also called the soul. This is what Jesus called the Father. Why? Because that piece of God that was created is identical to the soul within each of us.

How to Meditate?

First the simple basics, because meditation is very simple and not complicated at all. Then a more in depth explanation on the whys and why nots. There is no need to sit cross legged on the floor if it makes you uncomfortable. Just use a straight back chair so you can keep your back upright and straight.

- First, take a seat on the chair.
- Sit with your back up straight and your chin tucked comfortably down toward your chest.
- Place your hands on your thighs -- palms down.
- Put your feet next to one another, flat on the floor.
- Now close your eyes.
- Touch the tip of your nose with your finger, so you can see in the darkness exactly where you will put your eyes' full attention during the process of meditation. You want to be like an arrow of complete concentration, shooting deep into that darkness.
- How to breathe? When breathing, Don't expand your lungs outward on the inhale. Instead breathe in so the air goes downward as though filling the belly. When done correctly your belly area will move out and in as you breathe. This allows the diaphragm to move up and down. By not allowing the lungs to expand out and in, this helps you to use more lung capacity, without much effort.
- Now, a mantra or a word to help you focus. Choose AUM, OM, or AMEN. Each word effects the throat the same, as it is pronounced. As pronounced, it travels first touching the front of the roof of the mouth and moves back through to the throat. AMEN comes from AUM as the word moved and changed along the way, from India to the Middle East.

- The Key is to be so perfect in how you perform these instructions correctly, that in the end you want to literally feel like a rock anchored to the earth.

Now here is how you will put it all together in order of importance:

- Decide from the start that meditation will be done every day from this point forward. Meditate 20 minutes twice a day. Or for one hour per day, every day. I recommend the second one, plus having you make it a point to sit in meditation longer and longer. As this is a great way to really calm yourself during meditation and feel what it is like to rest beautifully in a super deep, very calm meditation. The longer you meditate, the deeper you go and the more you see for yourself, the benefits meditation has to offer. Not to mention the quicker you reach prefect results.
- Find a quiet place in the house where you will not be disturbed during meditation. Demand that your family and friends respect your peace and quiet time.
- Do not Play music, ocean sounds, bubbling brook sounds, while meditating. You want to discipline yourself, as these things work against you. Why? Because the idea is to turn off all sensual sensations (distractions from the five senses) going within the body.
- The goal of meditation is to become Self-Realized. You are looking for the true you your soul. This happens in the 6th dimension, not in this physical world or the 3rd dimension. You want to reach the Chamber of God or Genesis the point of all creation.
- Concentration on the point in the darkness, behind the tip of the nose is most important. Holding your concentration on this point is the key to your success. It's the point you will always return to and hold with all your attention, every time your mind wanders off.
- Hold your concentration while repeating your mantra word (MENTALLY). Repeat it slowly, over and over to yourself, with your full attention on it being pronounced properly. This means, not in a lazy way, as this bad habit is easy to become comfortable with and is a sign that you could be distracted, even to the point of falling asleep.
- Very important Your mind's thoughts are going to fight you every step of the way as you meditate, so be ready to fight back with alertness.
- You will fall asleep! The mind will be like a monkey and wander away, chasing after your thoughts and day dreams. You will be distracted by all types of body sensations. Even your eyes will look away from the tip of your nose. Even your mind will move from your head down to your belly and surprise you, in the sense that you never thought it was possible. Ignore all of these things. If you

want to ponder it after meditation, fine, but ignore everything during your meditation session.

- Want absolutely nothing from the process of meditation or you will fail at reaching self-realization. Meditation is not a process of wanting self-realization reaching out and grabbing it, like you do with things in life. God blesses you with it! Now know this. You are not going to take it. Because of the above statement. Learn to put yourself in a position of doing meditation for the sole purpose of doing the procedure correctly and letting God handle the rest. PUT IN THE time no matter how long it takes and the reward will come on its own. Like any journey, it starts with the first mile. So look at your journey as some place far off in the future. A place that you don't know how far away it is but in time you'll get there.

- Checking your posture. Every so often, as you meditate; you will check on your posture to be sure your back is straight up, chin is tucked down a bit, legs are together and hands remain palm side down on the thighs. Do this mentally without opening the eyes.

- Check the body to feel if you are tense anywhere. When you feel that you are, mentally relax the whole body and continue.

- Before meditating, know that you do not want to stuff yourself with food. Have one piece of fruit or a single slice of toast and water no coffee. Save that for later, as those heavy meals can make you tired, even though you may have just woke up from a night's sleep. Coffee can cause the mind to race. Always eat light about one hour before you meditate.

- You will fall asleep sometimes. It's okay! Once you've had that cat nap, straighten out your posture and continue. Understand that every night when you go to sleep your soul rests outside your physical body. It is always awake when the body sleeps.

Here's a final wrap up to put all of this simply together:

- Hold your concentration and return to it when the mind wanders for any reason.

- From time to time check over the body from head to toe for tension. When discovered -relax that spot and continue.

- Be distracted by nothing. When distracted, return to the place of concentration.

- Want nothing. Sit like a witness to nothing.

- Sit contently as you meditate.

- Do not become impatient. Know that Self-Realization is given to you, not taken.

- Make time to meditate for long periods of time. This is how you get to know your inner self.
- Stay dedicated to doing meditation.
- Extra help to become calm and concentrated -- breathing exercises to do before meditation.
- Do as much or as little as you want, but do some.
- Good luck.
- Next, Some things that might happen to you and when they do -- treat them as no big deal and move on continuing to meditate properly.

As stated above. You may notice your mind go from being where you are use to it being in the area of the head to say, your belly; as you breathe in and out in this area. This will shock you. Don't worry, as it just proves that you are a spiritual being, not the physical being you have come to know and rely on.

You may feeling a tingling feeling between your eyebrows. This is a stirring of the third eye. It is perfectly normal and something that you need to let go of and get back to the process of meditation.

In this area of the third eye, you might even feel a knocking. Like when one knocks on a door. This too is normal and nothing to get excited about. The first thing that might come to mind is where in the Bible it says: "Knock and it shall be opened to you."

This happened to me a short time before we entered the 6th dimension, as did all the above. Just know that this may not happen to you, as the consciousness is infinite and you may go through something very different. This is why we say to ignore all sensations as they may hinder your success. You may feel, while concentrating on the tip of the nose, like you are moving forward, downward, upward, backward in the darkness. Ignore it. As you relax, your body will twitch. It's okay and normal.

Your eyes may pull upward to the third eye in a very intense way. To the point that your whole face will feel distorted. Again, it's okay. Just let it happen no matter how long it takes to subside. When it does, just notice how much more calm and relaxed you feel when you focus back on the nose again.

All of a sudden, for no reason at all, your back will slowly straighten up without you needing to do anything. Just let it happen and notice how much better you feel.

Health Benefits of Transcendental Meditation

Many of us have observed how we, or others, appear to look older following a period of particular challenge in our lives, and now research is now indicating that stress is in fact a contributor to premature biological ageing. Although the exact mechanisms by which this occurs are not yet clear, what we do know is that the release of stress chemicals during the fight or flight response creates biological changes.

Recent research found that work-related exhaustion can have a harmful effect on critical DNA in the cells, shortening the length of sections called telomeres. This wearing effect has been linked to health problems such as Parkinson's, type 2 diabetes, cardiovascular disease and cancer, and whilst known to occur over time, the study suggests that anxiety and stress may accelerate this.

Research has also found that in addition to speeding up heart rate and increasing blood pressure, Prolonged and repeated production of the stress hormone adrenaline creates a constriction of blood vessels, which can lead to impairment of vision and hearing. Another study found that the mere anticipation of stress can increase signs of ageing on the cellular level.

The understanding that TM practice dissolves accumulated stress in the body explains how research indicates that the long term practice of TM can create a reversal of the biological ageing process (how old a person is physiologically). One study found that a group who had been practicing TM for more than five years were physiologically 12 years younger, and others practicing less than five years were physiologically five years younger than their chronological age. This was measured by reduction of blood pressure, and better near-point vision and auditory discrimination (effects of diet and exercise controlled for).

Asthma and Breathing

Our breath is affected by stress. The 'fight or flight' response causes us to take short sharp breaths in preparation for danger. The build-up of stress and the chronic activation of this response can mean we constantly breathe like this, only ever using the top third of our lungs, as if we were permanently hyperventilating. This leads to a poor exchange of oxygen and CO^2 in the bloodstream, depriving our bodies of both vital gases.

The physiological effect of a lack of CO^2 can make us feel 'spaced out' and can lead to panic attacks, insomnia, dizziness and extreme fatigue, while lack of oxygen can rob our organs and muscles of a proper blood flow. Hyperventilating also increases the heart rate, leading to palpitations and contributes to feelings of anxiety and being out of control. The stress response can also create strong physiological reactions that lead to airway constriction and changes in the immune system, which can worsen asthma symptoms. Recent research has found that certain areas of the brain cause worsening asthma symptoms when a person is under stress.

The improvements in our breathing, but also in asthma symptoms, and other respiratory problems as a result of practicing TM can be therefore understood as an effect of dissolving stress and reduced 'stress reactivity'. A study of data showed that both hospital admission and outpatient consultation rates were over 50% lower for subjects practising TM than norms or controls. Admissions were 73% less for respiratory disorders.

A few studies have indicated that regular practice of TM can lead to improvements in Patients with Bronchial Asthma, including reduced severity of symptoms, reduced airway resistance and less need for medication. One study found these improvements in the symptoms of 21 patients over six months, concluding that TM is a useful adjunct to treatment. Other research has indicated fewer upper respiratory tract infections, improvements in chronic bronchitis, and more efficient breathing and respiratory control.

Blood Pressure

Numerous research studies and reviews have concluded that 'stress' is a major independent risk factor for hypertension as well as coronary artery disease and cardiovascular mortality. The 'fight/flight' or stress response which is triggered by our reaction to life's challenges increases the heart rate. In cases of persistent hyper activation, this can to lead to chronically elevated blood pressure levels. Since stress is such a major factor with blood pressure problems, it is no surprise that TM, which reverses the stress response, can have a very significant impact, occasionally dramatic, on the problem.

Although research generally focuses on high blood pressure, which TM naturally reduces, this does not mean that in cases of low blood pressure it will also reduce. TM has its effect because it allows the body to gain very deep rest which activates the body's natural healing mechanisms, which only take effect when there is a problem to be solved. So if blood pressure is low it will tend to rise, if it is already at the correct level there will be no change. The experiences of thousands of meditators has shown this to be the case. Many studies have found that TM decreases blood pressure in hypertensive patients. A systematic review and metaanalysis of 107 published studies on stress reduction and high blood pressure found that TM practice significantly reduced both systolic and diastolic blood pressure, while other methods of meditation and relaxation, biofeedback, stress management or the usual health advice programmes did not produce significant effects. Effects were comparable to those commonly found with anti-hypertensive medication, but without adverse side-effects, and medication use was reduced. A second meta-analysis confirmed that TM leads to clinically important reductions in blood pressure. The authors conclude that sustained blood pressure changes like those produced by TM would be associated with substantially decreased risk of heart attack and stroke, the leading cause of world mortality.

Cancer

People who have cancer often find the physical, emotional, and social effects to be extremely challenging. Those who attempt to manage their resulting stress with risky behaviours such as smoking or drinking alcohol or who become more sedentary may have a poorer quality of life after cancer treatment. And some data suggests that patients who develop a sense of helplessness or hopelessness when stress becomes overwhelming may have a higher instance of negative outcomes.

The practice of TM, with its significant effect in reducing an individual's physiological stress levels indicated by scientific research, has produced a good amount of anecdotal evidence from sufferers pointing to its ability to improve, sometimes dramatically, the patient's coping ability, and therefore their experience of the process, and research has supported that TM has a positive impact on quality of life for breast cancer patients (Integrative Cancer Therapies).

But improving a patient's experience and coping power in the cancer recovery process is not the only potential benefit of TM's powerful dissolving of the body's accumulated stress. Evidence from experimental studies also suggests that stress hormones can stimulate a tumour's ability to grow and spread, whilst the practice of TM has been found to reduce stress hormones, and therefore should have potentially greater significance for patients than simply increasing coping power.

Ayurveda ('the science of life') the world's oldest natural healthcare system in continuous use for more than 5000 years, has much to say on the potential of its natural approaches, such as the TM technique which is at its heart, for awakening nature's healing intelligence.

How Transcendental Meditation is Different

A common mistake made by the casual observer is to think that all meditation is basically the same. It is now clearly shown by scientific research that the various techniques of meditation differ not only in the actual mental process being used, but also in the very different effects that have been measured in the brain and their effect on our lives. So how is transcendental meditation different?

In essence, there is one fundamental difference between TM and other approaches: Most meditation aims to control or train the mind by a way of thinking. Transcendence, on the other hand, involves no concentration, control, or training. (It is counter-productive to try to force the mind to go somewhere it already wants to go naturally!). TM allows the mind to go beyond surface level thinking towards silence (the source of thought) and concentration, focus and control as well as freedom and creativity are the spontaneous results.

A recent review of research has suggested three main categories of meditation:

- Focused Attention or concentration techniques (e.g. Zen, Qi gong, Vipassana) require effort to sustain controlled attention on an object, and therefore are characterised by high frequency activity in the front and core of the brain.

- Open Monitoring includes mindfulness-based techniques, in which all experiences are allowed to pass through awareness without manipulation or control, but the mind is generally being trained to return to the present moment by using an object, breath, or body as an anchor. These are characterised by theta activity primarily in the front of the brain.
- Automatic Self-Transcending (AST) involves neither concentration nor training the mind. Automatic means innocence is the key here. Evaluation, control or manipulation will leave you caught up in thinking and prevent transcending. AST includes TM, and the occasional expert in other techniques. It describes any technique which transcends (goes beyond) the steps of the meditation practice itself. Alpha brain waves (characteristic of reduced mental activity and relaxation) permeate the whole brain, which receives more oxygen. Increased blood flow to the front (which is coordinating activity) while the core of the brain is more quiet, indicates alertness in the midst of deep rest, the state of transcendental or pure consciousness (pure silence!).

So is Transcendental Meditation the best?

Each meditation technique has its own benefits. The first two categories use the conscious, surface level of the mind, training the mind to produce specific outcomes. TM, however, is the most effective technique for transcending, which means 'going beyond' this relatively surface level of thought to experience its source. From here we spontaneously return to activity with the dynamic power of nature's silent, restful alertness which then supports all our thought, speech and action (experienced briefly as the 'zone' in sport) and thereby produce a potentially much greater range of mental, physical and spiritual benefits.

Meta-analyses (statistical analysis of multiple research studies) have found that TM is more effective than other meditation or relaxation techniques in producing a range of results. Examples include:

- Reducing anxiety.
- Increasing self-actualisation.
- Decreasing blood pressure.
- Reducing addiction.

How does Transcendental Meditation Differ from Mindfulness?

The purpose of mindfulness, deriving from Buddhist traditions, is gently training the mind to be in the present moment. Whilst superficially appearing similar, TM and mindfulness are actually quite different. Rather than returning the attention to the breath, body or other objects, it is the use of a specific mantra, or sound, in TM which liberates rather than trains the mind, allowing it to settle effortlessly into a silence more profound than the present moment.

Increased mindfulness is just one of the many spontaneous effects of TM, as indicated by research: A 3-month randomised controlled trial found that those practising TM reported significantly greater increases in mindfulness than waitlist participants.

The full practice of meditation in the Yoga tradition was prevalent in India before and during the life of the Buddha. In this practice, the meditation itself is preceded and nourished by mindfulness in the form of Asana (yoga postures) and Pranayama (breathing techniques) when, most importantly, attention on first body and then breath create a state of Pratyahara, movement of attention inwards, away from the world's distractions.

The practice of meditation that follows is then, if properly applied, a simple, effortless and automatic continuation of the flow of attention towards peaceful, blissful silence, like a river flowing spontaneously towards the ocean. This understanding of effortless meditation was revived in India in the 1950s by Maharishi Mahesh Yogi as transcendental meditation.

Self-Inquiry Meditation

The process of Self-inquiry is so simple that it can be explained in a few words. One traces the root of one's thoughts back to the I-thought, from which all other thoughts arise and diverge. This is initiated by the question "Who am I?" or similar questions about one's true identity.

All our thoughts are based directly or indirectly on the thought of the self. Our thoughts consist of two components: a subjective factor — I, me or mine — and an objective factor— a state, condition or object with which we are involved — our own body and mind or external circumstances like our relationships, possessions or activities. We get caught in the object portion and fail to look within to see our true nature apart from these external conditioning influences.

The result is that the pure I or I-in-itself remains unknown to us. All that we call ourselves is but a conglomerate "I am this" or "this is mine," with the subject confused with an object. Our self becomes a self-image, a subject in the guise of an object, in which our intrinsic nature is lost, along with our dignity as a conscious being. We become a mere name and form, a commodity in the outer world to be used and exploited. Self-inquiry consists of detaching from the object portion to discover the pure Subject, so that we can become liberated from all external limitations.

The truth is that we don't know who we really are. What we call our Self is only some thought, emotion or sensation that we are temporarily identified with. We are trapped in ideas that we are happy or sad, good or bad, foolish or wise, but do not know the Self who experiences these changing qualities. Our lives are shrouded in ignorance about our true nature, starting with our bodily identity, the idea that we are no more than this changing physical vesture. As long as we don't question this process we must come to sorrow.

However, Self-inquiry does not mean merely to repeat the question "Who am I?" over and over again in our minds. This becomes an exercise in mental activity that breeds fatigue. It means searching for our true Self in all that we do, which is more a matter of observation than analysis, looking to the Self that is behind our various activities of breathing, eating, feeling, thinking and acting. Other questions can be helpful like "What am I?" or "Who is the experiencer?," or "Who is the seer?." Any type of self-introspection, in which we try to look dispassionately at who we are and the results of our actions, moves us in this direction.

Self-inquiry requires that we have a fundamental doubt about who we are that rejects all outer identifications. It is as if one had amnesia and didn't know who one was and had to give full attention to the matter before anything else could be done. Self-inquiry is not an intellectual or a psychological inquiry but an inquiry with one's entire energy and attention. It requires a full and one-pointed concentration, not interrupted by the intrusion of other thoughts.

True Self-inquiry is not just questioning the limitation of our outer identity, like our family, political or religious affiliations — whether one is a wife, a father, a Christian, Hindu or communist. It questions our internal identity as an embodied being and as a mind. It does not stop short with some general identity as a human, cosmic or spiritual being but rejects any formation of thought. It directs us back to the pure "I" that has no identity with any form of objectivity, physical or mental, that is in the world but not of it. The true Self is not only beyond human distinctions, it is beyond all conceivable divisions of time and space, name and form, birth and death. It is beyond all experience as the experiencer or observer of all.

The thought current naturally moves back to the Self to the extent that we do not preoccupy our minds with outside stimulation. The problem is that the senses present so many distractions that it is difficult to look within. Self-inquiry means to constantly question and try to reverse this process of extroversion, holding our awareness in the heart.

Self-inquiry leads us ultimately to the experience of the Absolute in which the phenomenal world becomes little more than a mirage of the mind and senses. It goes far beyond the discovery of some greater self, human or creative potential. It is called the direct way to the Absolute.

Self-Inquiry and Other Meditational Practices

Self-inquiry, it should be noted, is a kind of mental activity, though of a special nature.

It is not an attempt to suppress thought or to hold the mind in a blank or empty state, which can be another trap that prevents real transformation. Self-inquiry does not teach that all thought is bad but, in fact, that one form of thinking is necessary for liberation. It teaches us to use the mind in the right way, which is to turn it into a tool of inquiry. Self-inquiry requires much thoughtfulness, particularly in its preliminary phases, and the development of a strong mental discipline. Unless we have resolved our problems through deep examination it is useless, not to mention impossible, to stop the mind from thinking.

One may ask how Self-inquiry, a mental activity, can empty or silence the mind? Does not mental activity increase mental activity? It is not possible for the mind to be empty if its contents have not been released. Mental activity springs from a source, the "I-thought." We must go to the root of something to change it. This is to return to the I-thought in order to go beyond all other thoughts. Holding to the I-thought destroys all other thoughts.

Hence Self-inquiry is not a kind of passive mindfulness in which we focus on being aware of something, like our breath, hands or an activity that we may be doing. Self-inquiry does not say "Be aware of your breath" but, rather, "Who is breathing?" or "Who is really alive?" It does not say "Be mindful of your body," but rather asks "Are you the body?"

Similarly, Self-inquiry is not a form of concentration, in which we try to concentrate on one object, like a mantra, to the exclusion of all others. It is concentration on the Self where our attention automatically returns whatever else we may try to do. We cannot completely concentrate on anything else unless we first know ourselves. Otherwise the I-thought must arise and break the continuity of our concentration. Rather than fighting the I-thought and trying to return to an object of concentration, Self-inquiry concentrates on the I-thought to put an end to other thoughts.

Self-inquiry is also not an attempt to be good or to make ourselves better. It is questioning the reality of the entity who we think is either good or bad, can either improve or degenerate. It questions our efforts to be this or that and says that without knowing ourselves, without eliminating the root of the ego, it is of no lasting benefit to try to become anything, however great or noble.

Above all Self-inquiry is not an ordinary mental activity, a form of philosophical speculation or psychological analysis. It is not seeking any mental answer and has no conceptual result. While Self-inquiry leads to the absolute truth, which can be called the pure I or Self, the name is only a pointer. One can call it God, knowledge, enlightenment, Buddha or whatever one likes but it is not a state defined according to an idea, or in which mental recognition can occur. Self-inquiry is questioning of the validity of all entities and conclusions created by the mind. This does not mean that practices like mindfulness, ethical disciplines, mantra, pranayama or the study of scriptures do not have their place, but that these are supportive to Self-inquiry or an alternative line of approach. To follow ethical disciplines, to place the body in a comfortable position, to deepen the breath, to withdraw the mind from sensory stimulation, to develop concentration and other yogic practices, should be done, but we should not stop there but proceed to Self-inquiry. Only rare individuals can proceed directly to Self-inquiry and even they can benefit by such preliminary practices.

The Practice of Self-Inquiry

Self-inquiry can be done at all times, places and circumstances. It does not require knowledge of special yoga techniques. It does not require that we otherwise try to overtly change ourselves or what we are doing. It only requires that we place our attention on the source from which thought naturally springs. This, however, is one of the most difficult of all things because it requires control of the wavering and fickle mind. Yet there are several things that can help promote it.

Self-inquiry is done most easily when we are sitting alone, particularly in nature. The outer nature is the door to the inner nature. It provides the space and peace that allows the mind to return to its source. In nature, apart from our personal involvements, we can more easily inquire into who we really are, into not only the meaning of human life but that of cosmic existence.

We can practice Self-inquiry when we are around other people, but this requires more effort because social contact pulls the mind outward. It is important therefore to reduce our outer activities and social contacts to aid in Self-inquiry. Generally in India Self-inquiry is not done in a group setting, in a standardized manner or according to a specific course of practice. It is mainly done on an individual basis, though communion between practitioners is encouraged as is specific instruction from the teacher.

To practice Self-inquiry while we are engaged in action we can call to mind the inquiry "Who is the doer?" In this way we will not let our actions dominate our awareness. This in fact gives us better skill in action because it removes any ego distortions from what we are attempting to do. Perhaps the easiest way to approach to change. One's power of seeing remains constant through the various objects seen.

Second, one discriminates the seer from the sense organs. In this instance the mind is the seer and the senses are the seen. There are several senses and each one varies in acuity but the seer of the senses is constant and not altered by their fluctuations. For example, the seer of the eye is not tarnished by any impairments in the eye, like loss of visual acuity.

Third, one discriminates between the seer and mental states. The self is the seer and the mind is the seen.Thoughts and feelings continually change but their seer, if we look deeply, remains the same. Our seeing as a child and as an adult is the same seeing, not only of external objects but of our internal thoughts and feelings.

Fourth, one discriminates between the seer and the ego, between the pure-I or higher Self and and the lower self, the I identified with body, emotion or thought. We learn to observe ourselves and our personal limitations, as external forms like our house or our car. We see the ego as various mental conditions but not the true Self that is beyond the mind. The pure Self devoid of external associations can then shine forth. One then strives to abide in that state of pure awareness. And in this process one is to negate external objects as not the Self or not I. Then one can negate internal thoughts and feelings, including the ego itself. Whatever one can perceive as an object externally or internally is not the Self who is the witness of all.

How to do Self Inquiry Meditation?

- Step 1: To begin the practice of self-inquiry, sit for meditation as usual. If you don't already have a regular practice, just sit quietly and allow the mind to settle naturally. Don't attempt to focus your mind or manipulate your experience, just rest as awareness itself.

- Step 2: After 10 or 15 minutes introduce the question "Who am I?" Drop the question into the stillness of your being like a pebble into a still forest pool. Let it send ripples through your meditation, but don't attempt to figure it out.

- Step 3: When the pond is tranquil again, drop in another pebble and see what happens. Set aside any conceptual answers, such as "I am a child of God" or "I am consciousness" or "I am a spiritual being of light," and come back to the question. Though true at a certain level, these answers will not satisfy your hunger for spiritual sustenance.

- Step 4: Instead of "Who am I?" you may prefer asking, "Who is thinking this thought? Who is seeing through these eyes right now?"

- Step 5: For the practice of self-inquiry to work its magic, you must recognize at some level that the word I, though superficially referring to the body and mind, actually points to something much deeper.

- Step 6: Let your inquiry be earnest but effortless, without tension or anxiety. Here's a hint: You definitely won't find the answer in the file folders of spiritual beliefs you've amassed over the years, so look elsewhere, in your actual, present experience.

- Step 7: Eventually, the question "Who am I?" reveals the answer, not as a thought or a particular experience but as a vibrant, timeless presence that underlies and infuses every experience.

Yoga and Jainism

Yoga and Meditation have been the fundamental practice of spirituality in Jainism. It has been a core spiritual practice for all Tirthankaras. All twenty-four Tirthankaras were human beings, they all practiced different physical yoga postures and deep meditation for several years to attain a state of perfect enlightenment and self-realization.

Mahavir swami, at age of 30 renounced the worldly life and spent twelve and half years in yoga and deep meditation. During this period, he progressed spiritually and conquered desires, feelings, attachments and destroyed four Ghati (deluding) karma and attained enlightenment or Keval-Jnan, while in Goduhikasana (milking posture).

Yoga and Meditation helps us realize the true nature of our soul. Jain religion is based Bhava (internal reflection) and our spiritual progress is towards reducing of our vices or Kashaya. Meditation can help us grow spiritually while finding inner peace, inner calmness, purpose of life and equanimity.

Archeological evidence and the study of ancient scripture suggest that Yoga and Meditation were practiced in ancient India as early as 3000 BC. There are several Aacharyas who have contributed towards development of Yoga and Meditation in Jainism.

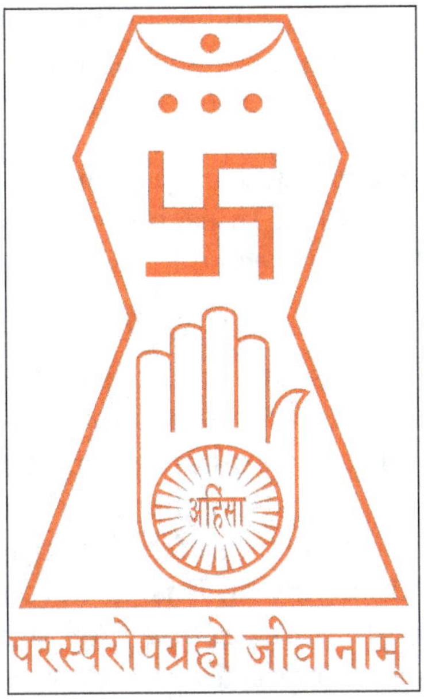

There are two differing interpretaions of the meaning of the word Yoga: According to Patanjali Rishi, one needs to stop thoughts and move inwards. However, one has to also recognize that the cessation of the activities of mind, speech and body does not in itself lead to immediate inner peace and tranquility as our mental state remains disturbed due to the effect of the kashayas (passions of anger, greed, ego, deceit) which are within us. Just as we cannot control the wind, in the same way we cannot control our thoughts which remain free and take us here and there and everywhere in the shortest of moments.

Acharya Hemachandra has therefore concluded that true spiritual practice is not to stop our thoughts, but instead to focus on getting rid of the negativities, the vices which are within us. It is the negative actions which we do as a result of the fruition of our kashayas which gives rise to new karmas. We have to stop yoga of this negative type and rid ourselves of these negativities. Mind, speech and body are only a conduit but ones which can take us either to bliss (moksha) or to hell. They are the vehicles to cross the ocean. So how can we even talk about quieting these activities? No, it is their very nature – mind's nature is to think, body's nature is to act and speech's action is to speak.

Can we ever stop our thoughts? Can we stop the wind? Just as we cannot get rid of the wind, so our thoughts, our speech and our bodily actions cannot be stopped. The speech and words directed at us by others, who is it that is taking heed of these words and accepting them? It is the kashayas within us which are attracted by and hold on to these words, will not forget them and then lead us to react to what was said by the other person. Just as the camera captures a photo, in the same way our kashayas capture that which we see and hear. It is important to remember that we should try not to keep these resulting imprints stored inside us. We need to keep ourselves 'light' and vigilant. Then when we see or hear something, there will be clarity rather than negativity. Otherwise even during meditation, we will visualise and recall only the negativities residing within us.

So what should our yoga be? According to Jain philosophy, there are 4 types of dhyan – Artha, Raudra, Dharma and Shukla. In each of these 4 types of dhyan, there is an intensity of focus and concentration directed in a certain way.

Artha dhyan – Here the concentration is inward looking, focusing on looking at ourselves and on the unhappiness and sadness we are experiencing which arise from our own actions and perceptions. We have forgotten our true nature and our self respect. Why accept negativities directed at us by others and make ourselves unhappy? One day spend time to reflect from morning until night and observe what happens inside you if someone insults you. Who is connecting with this insult? No one else but you! The person has not forced this insult on to you! It is up to you whether you want to receive and ingest this insult. It is open to you to refuse! For instance, if you go to the market and there you see a lot of unneeded items for sale, do these items end up in your home without effort? No, not unless you take the step to buy them and bring them home, which only you can do.

In the very same way you are standing in this worldly market– when sadness comes in then consider who has 'bought' this. Remember it does not come free, it requires 'money'. Our normal reaction is to listen to what has come our way, think about it, reflect on it and make it into something 'juicy' and then store it within you. This is just waste of energy. This is artha dhyan where the intense concentration is directed on yourself and your needs.

- Raudra Dhyan: On the other hand the focus of raudra dhyan is on blaming others or external things. He did this, he did that, he did not do this, he does not listen, it is hot, so cold, so much sun, so much rain, such people the list is endless. Those who become saddened by looking at others is raudra dhyan. There is no passion to do any good work, just to keep on complaining and only on thinking about how to put others down. If Duryadhan had not had this intense concentration of raudra dhyan, then he would not have been empowered to humiliate Draupadi.

- Dharma Dhyan: To see good in this world and appreciate all is to nurture dharma dhyan. If our concentration is on looking at what is good in the world, have a desire to be part of this goodness and try to walk on this path of goodness – all these are dharma dhyan.

- Shukla Dhyan: All the negativities, the goodness is all within you, not outside. This is reality. Everything externally is neither good nor bad. It is how you conceive everything. Everything is so transparent; there is no distinction between inside and outside. This is shukla dhyan and arises only after keval gyan is achieved.

To achieve both worldly bondage and liberation, requires intense concentration and focus. In our spiritual practices we need to move away from artha dhyan and raudra dhyan and move towards dharma dhyan. Shukla dhyan is still too distant for us. Righteous meditation is of an auspicious type and Jainism holds that liberation can only be achieved through meditation or Shukla Dhyana. It is important to know both the sides, so we can have the awareness and guide ourselves to the righteous meditation.

The twelve bhavnas (reflections) in Jainism are a mental exercise in introspection and are intended to create a greater awareness of the need for detachment and constant devotion to religion. The twelve kinds of reflections are:

- Anitya Bhävanä (Impermanence): Reflection that everything in this world is transient. Good or Bad, nothing is forever.

- Asharan Bhävanä (Helplessness): Reflection that there is nothing or no person in this world under whom I can take shelter or protection except for my soul, path of religion and my virtues.

- Samsär Bhävanä (Endless cycles of birth and death): Reflection on the endless cycles of births and deaths which bring in endless suffering and misery. One should feel tired of the trans-migratory existence and seek for remedies of escape from fetters of Karmas.

- Ekatva Bhävanä (Solitude of the soul): Reflection that I am my Savior. Thinking that - I am born alone and shall have to die alone; none can save me from transmigration, except myself, my religious convictions, my virtues, and my pious life. This frees us from attachments and brings equanimity of mind.
- Anyatva Bhävanä (Your body and soul are separate entity): Reflection that the soul is distinct from the body. This body is perishable, and all acquired relations/things because of the body are not mine. I am soul, which is not perishable and only soul is capable of attaining liberation.
- Ashuchi Bhävanä (Impure state of the body): Reflection on the uncleanness and impurities of the body. This reflection helps discard our attachments to our body, and engage in self-discipline, renunciation, and spiritual endeavors.
- Äsrava Bhävanä (Influx of Karma): Reflection on the influx of Karmas which leads to distress and misery in life. Any cause such as wrong belief (Mithyätva) or passions (Kashäya) that create the inflow of Karmas should be discarded.
- Samvar Bhävanä (Stopping the Influx of Karma): Reflection on the need for stoppage or influx of Karmas. One must carry out all the activities with the intention to reduce or stop new bondage of Karma.
- Nirjarä Bhävanä (Eradication of Karma): Reflection on the methods of shedding away the Karmas. Raising our spirituality through various means to shed our Karmas.
- Loka-svabhäva Bhävanä (Ever changing universe): Reflection on the nature of the universe, soul, and matter, and about the nature of the other substances.
- Bodhidurlabh Bhävanä (A rare chance to be enlightened): Reflection that religious instruction is difficult to obtain. It is difficult to attain right faith, right knowledge and right conduct, as many would be indulging in the enjoyment of worldly pleasures which attract us most and make us forget altogether the need to secure enlightenment for the soul which is of vital importance for its liberation.
- Dharma Bhavna (True religion is an excellent shelter): Reflection on what has been taught by the our tirthankaras. Such contemplation induces devotion to the principles of ahimsa, truth, honesty, celibacy, humility, and equanimity which form the integral parts of the teachings of Jainism. With such contemplation again and again, the mind will be turned inward, fully restrained and no attachment.

A constant reminder of these twelve Bhävanäs expands our understanding of the life's situations/events and helps us in transitioning from non-virtuous to virtuous meditation.

Jain Meditation

In Jainism meditation has been the central practice since a long stretch of time. Meditation or Dhyana is regarded as the supreme penance out of the 12 types of penances. It requires higher purity and detachment from the external things to reach the highest form of meditation called Shukla Dhyana or Perfect Meditation. In the end of Shukla Dhyana the practitioner attains Absolute Knowledge, Absolute Perception, and experiences Absolute Bliss. In Jainism, such state of a soul is called Kevala Gyana and Kevala Darshana. But in order to achieve this state of perfect purity the seeker has to go through the 14 Stages of Spiritual Development. In the entire practice, the practitioner strives to be just a Knower & Seer.

Right Knowledge

Before the seeker begins his practice he should have the Right Knowledge of reality. In other words, he should be familiar and should have faith on the principles like Anekantvada, Soul and Matter, Substance and its modes. Thus the seeker realizes his goal and the way to achieve it.

Meditation begins with Right Knowledge, the knowledge of Soul, Matter (Atoms), and other four substances like Medium of Motion, Medium of Rest, Space and Time. All the six substances should be understood with their Permanence, Emergence and Cessation attributes. After knowing this and having faith in these core principles of Jainism the seeker realizes his/her real self and distinguishes his /her real self from the non-self substances. The truth is, one's own soul is completely independent from all other souls as well as from other substances like Matter, Motion, Rest, Space and Time. Every soul is independent and every atom is independent. All the six substances are independent from each other. The truth is multi-dimensional. It is impossible to express the truth in one view point.

Cognitive Function

The basic attribute of a soul is Cognitive Function. Every substance has its own attributes and they have intrinsic relation. For example, the attributes of matter are Color, Sound, Touch, Form, Taste, Smell and Material Energy. The attributes of a soul are Knowledge, Perception, Bliss and Spiritual Energy. The soul is fully conscious, formless, all knowing and all perceiving substance. There are infinite souls in the cosmos and all are independent from each other. Together, the knowing and perceiving capability of each soul is called Cognitive Function or Upayoga. Knowing both the Special and General attributes of a substance is called the Cognitive Function of a soul. The Cognitive Function can also be termed as attention or Psyche. It is the basic attribute of a soul and the self realization can be gained by being in tune with it.

Constant Vigilance

In Jainism, constant vigilance means meditation. The seeker or the true sage strives to keep his/her cognition (Upayoga) on the true nature of the soul. In every moment the seeker tries not to give up the contemplation of, "I am an independent soul, I was never born and am never going to cease, I am formless, eternal, possessing the qualities of Infinite Knowledge and Perception. I am free from this body; I have no smell nor color, no weight nor form."

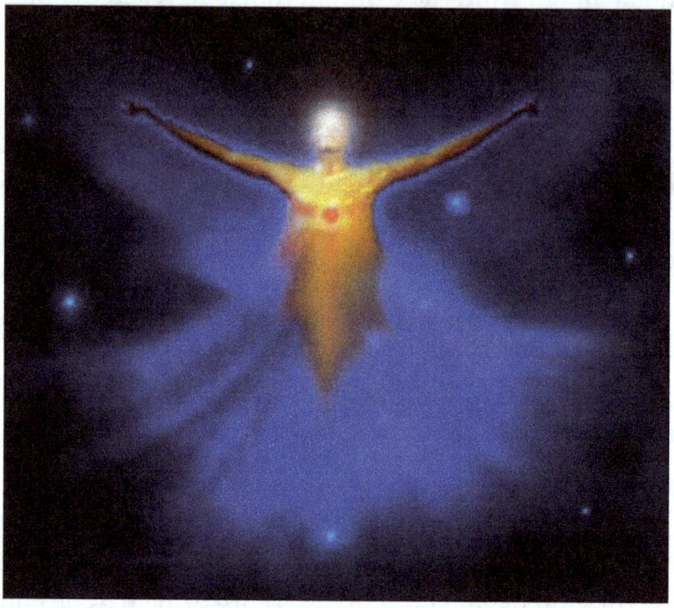

There is mention of three types of regulations in Jainism. The three regulations are also known as Three Guptis. These are, Regulation of Mind, Regulation of Speech, and Regulation of Bodily activity. The practice of three regulations is the first step for the seeker. To reach the higher stages of meditation the seeker must master the three regulations. The three regulations cannot be practiced fully without taking the Five Great Vows. Thus the monk who has taken five vows becomes potentially viable for righteous meditation. The mundane being who hasn't taken the five vows can still practice Samayika. Samayika is a term used for a short period meditation. In Samayika one stops his/her daily activities for 48 minutes, sits motionless and concentrates upon the pure nature of a soul.

To remain vigil, it is important to reduce the bodily activities as well as the activities of mind and speech. At this point when all these three kind of activities ceases the seeker can feel the consciousness (chetana). In the higher stages of meditation such feeling and bliss can be felt even while walking, taking meal, or doing some bodily activity. It is written in the scriptures that Lord Mahavir, the 24th Jain Tirthankara was always vigil even while walking or having meal. He was ceaselessly conscious at every moment of the day and night, total vigilance in the sixth step, and Samadhi, the seventh step of the meditative path.

Changing the lifestyle is very important in order to reach the higher stages of meditation. Taking up the five vows helps in changing lifestyle. The monk who has taken the great five vows easily gets rid of the activity of mind, speech and body, but only when if he/she has the true knowledge and faith and has only goal of attaining liberation. On the other hand the one who lives mundane life and has all sensual pleasures finds difficult to practice meditation for a longer duration because the mundane thoughts keeps coming in the mind and the concentration on the soul becomes difficult. So, changing the lifestyle, with true knowledge, under the guidance of a true spiritual guru, plays an important role in spiritual progress. Though there are 12 types of minor vows for the mundane beings. Practicing these vows the mundane soul can progress towards purity and in the end becomes able to take up five great vows.

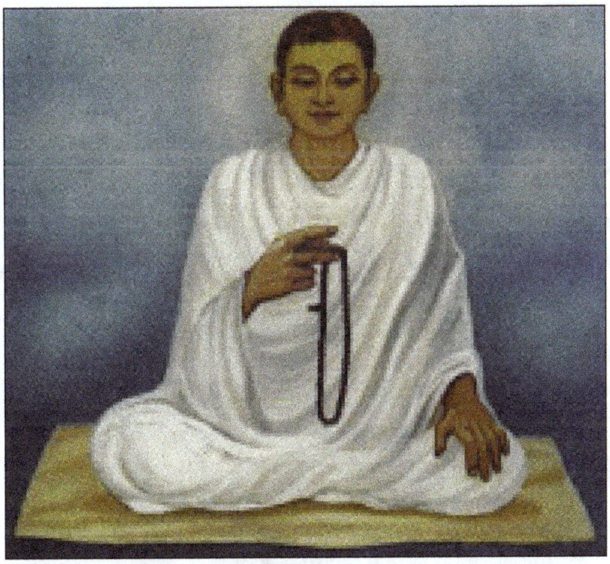

A picture depicts a Jain Layman practicing Samayik.

Dharma Dhyana and Shukla Dhyana

According to Jainism, we all are always in meditation wherever our cognition is focused, whether it is virtuous or non-virtuous. To pay attention or to focus the cognition to particular object, or thoughts is meditation. There are four types of meditation, Wrathful, Sorrowful, Righteous and Spiritual Meditation. The first two are non-virtuous meditations because they cause karma bondage; the latter two are virtuous meditations as they prevent the influx of karma particles as well as destroy all karma.

Dharma Dhyana or Virtuous Meditation is the root of Spiritual Meditation (Shukla Dhyana) and Omniscience. In Virtuous Meditation one strives to keep his/her cognition fixed on the pure form of the soul and also tries to minimize mental choices and volitions. When choices and volitions arise then the meditation shifts to Sorrowful or Wrathful, thus binds karma. To think about mundane world, bodily pleasure or hurting someone is Sorrowful and Wrathful meditation.

Shukla Dhyana or Spiritual Meditation is the result of Dharma Dhyana. The aspirant starts practicing Dharma Dhyana when he/she renounces the world. The aim of

Dharma Dhyana is to achieve the stage of Shukla Dhyana. Shukla Dhyana occurs in the end of the 12th stage when the soul destroys the Conduct Deluding Karma (Charitra Mohaniya Karma) and gains unprecedented stability and bliss. Now this stability of spiritual meditation never ceases and takes the soul to the second stage of Shukla Dhyana and here the soul destroys the remaining three karma namely Knowledge Obscuring, Perception Obscuring and Destructing Karma and enters the state of Kevala or Omniscience. Omniscience or Kevala, in other words can be defined as constant spiritual awareness. Shukla Dhyana, after it starts helps the practitioner destroy all the four destructive karma within 48 minutes.

In Dharma Dhyana the aspirant strived to be constant aware about his/her true self. The aspirant was constant vigil and very careful on his activities of mind, speech and body. The more vigil he remained the more purity he gained and the karma became weak. As a result permanence awareness and bliss manifested within that is called Shukla Dhyana. In Dharma Dhyana the monk feels the soul and its pure bliss in broken parts but in Shukla Dhyana, the bliss, experience becomes intact, unbroken and whole and keeps feeling the infinite bliss, infinite knowledge and infinite perception forever.

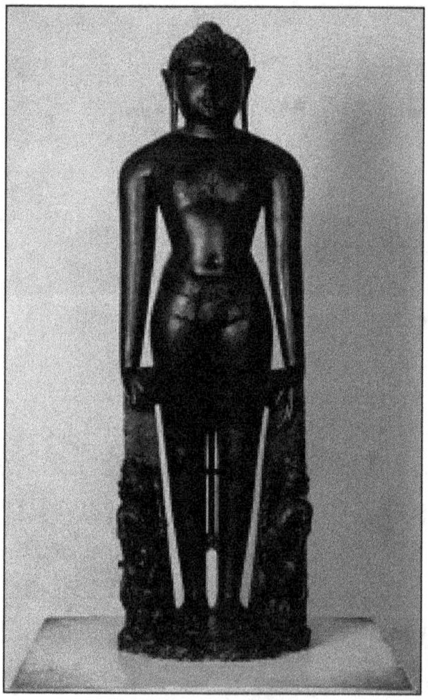

A Jain Tirthankara in Kayotsarga posture.

Kayotsarga and Dhyana

Kayotsarga and Dhyana (Meditation) are the most important austerities. Kayotsarga means steadiness of the mind, speech and body. Once the activities of mind, body and speech ceases the soul can be experienced. Kayotsarga is the first step of meditation. It is important to have these three types of bodily activities to be ceased before the pure consciousness can be felt. Kayotsarga is very important for the beginners. Kayotsarga is related with body while meditation is related with soul. Kayotsarga is one kind of yogic posture and can be practiced in sitting, laying or standing posture. After practicing kayotsarga and stopping all kind of physical activities, meditation becomes easy to practice and there comes moments in which the true soul and pure bliss can be felt.

Fourteen Stages of Spiritual Development

Jainism acknowledges that the soul advances to its liberated stage in various steps, called Gunasthan or "The Stages of Spiritual Development". Through these fourteen stages of development, the soul gradually frees itself, firstly from the worst, then from the less bad and finally from all kinds of karma, and manifests the innate qualities of knowledge, belief and conduct in a more and more perfect form. Here we will take a glance at each stage of spiritual development. Dharma Dhyana or Righteous Meditation plays an important role in climbing each stage and the external austerities like fasting, giving up tasty food etc helps in supporting meditation. The goal is to reach the highest type of meditation (Shukla Dhyana) and liberation.

- The stage of wrong believer: The lowest stage with ignorance, delusion, and with intense attachments and aversions. This is the normal condition of all souls involved in the mundane world and is the starting point of spiritual evolution.
- The stage of one who has a slight taste of right belief: Indifference to reality with occasional vague memory of spiritual insight.
- The stage of mixed belief: Fleeting moments of curiosity towards understanding reality.
- The stage of one who has true belief but has not yet self-discipline: Awareness of reality with trust developed in the right view, combined with willingness to practice self-discipline. The soul may be able to subdue the four passions namely anger, pride, deceit and greed.
- The stage of partial self-control: At this stage the right view and discipline starts to develop. The soul now begins to observe some of the rules of right conduct with a view to perfect itself. With the discipline of introductory or minor vows, the soul starts on the process of climbing spiritual ladder.
- The stage of complete self-discipline, although sometimes brought into wavering through negligence: Major vows taken up with firm resolve to control passions. There may be failures due to lack of full control over passions and carelessness.
- The stage of self-control without negligence: At this stage the self discipline and knowledge develops more. Intense practice of vows assisted in better self-control and virtually replaced carelessness with spiritual vigilance and vigor.

- The stage of one in whom the passions are still occurring in a gross form: The stage of one in whom the passions are still occurring in a gross form. Closer to perfect self-control over actions, higher control over mind, thought and passions with the soul ready for reduction of the effects of conduct-deluding karma.
- The stage of higher control over removal of passions and elimination of conduct-deluding karma begins.
- The stage of one in whom the passions occur in a subtle form but complete elimination of all passions except for subtle degree of attachment.
- The stage of one who has suppressed every passion but still does not possess omniscience. Suppressed passions and lingering conduct-deluding karma may rise to drag the soul to lower stages; fleeting experiences of equanimity.
- The stage of who has annihilated every passion. This is the point of no return. All passions as well as conduct-deluding karma are eliminated. Permanent internal peace achieved. No new bondage from this point onwards.
- The stage of omniscience with physical body. The all Destructive karma eliminated and Arihant stage reached. The perfected soul is still trapped in the physical body due to presence of remaining Non-Destructive Karma. The Lord Arihant now preaches others the path of liberation and helps seekers showing the path to cross the ocean of rebirths and reach the safe shore.
- The stage of omniscience without physical body. Siddha Stage reached and the purest soul after destroying the remaining non-destructive karmas attains Nirvana and reaches the abode of the liberated soul. Now the soul is free from the cycle of births and deaths and enjoys infinite bliss.

Meditation Techniques

Sorrowful Meditation

The Sanskrit word aarta means sorrow. The thought-activity caused by an outburst and intensity of sorrow is sorrowful meditation. It is of four types:

- Distaste Related (anishtasamyog janya) sorrowful meditation is persistent thoughts and worry about the removal of disagreeable orients, situations or events.
- Attachment related (ishtaviyoga janya) sorrowful meditation is the constant feelings of anguish an the loss of some agreeable object or person, such as wealth, spouse or child, and the preoccupation to recover the lost objects.
- Suffering related (vedana janya) sorrowful meditation is the feeling of impatience, grief and agony in the face of disease, sickness, etc., and the worry about its going away.

- Desires related (nidaanaj) sorrowful meditation is having persistent desires for future sensual pleasures and comforts.

Inclement Meditation

The sanskrit word rudra means inclement (harsh, lacking mercy). The meditation involving inclement thoughts is called inclement meditation. Based on the cause, inclement meditation has been divided into four types:

- Violence enchantment (himsa anand) inclement meditation involves thoughts of enchantment (delight) generated by teasing, hurting and/or killing animals. Cruel, angry, immoral, nonreligious and passionate people indulge in such meditation. Violence-enchantment meditation also includes contemplation about revenge, planning to beat or kill someone and enjoying visions of deadly war scenes.
- Untruth enchantment (mrisha anand) inclement meditation is thought involving false imagination stained with sinful intentions. A person with this type of meditation takes delight in a variety of intentions and alternatives based on untruth.
- Stealing enchantment (chaurya anand) inclement meditation involves thoughts of ways to steal and misappropriate other's wealth or beautiful things.
- Pleasure preservation (vishaya samrakshan) inclement meditation is contemplation about schemes of enjoyment of sensual pleasures and of accumulation of material wealth and the means of material comforts.

Sorrowful and inclement meditations hinder spiritual uplift, They obscure the attributes of soul. They cause the natural disposition of self to disappear and initiate corrupt dispositions. Both these meditations are inauspicious and lead to undesirable destinations. They are not related to spiritual advancement in any manner.

Spiritual Meditation

The concentration achieved by an immaculate mind is spiritual meditation. It consists of four states: Multi aspect (prathakatva savitarka savichar), single aspect (ekatva savitarka avichar), subtle activity (sookshma kriya apratipaati) and absorption in self (vyuparat kriya nivarti).

Multi aspect spiritual meditation is performed by an aspirant who has scriptural knowledge and who is attempting to attain the spiritual stages of subsidence or destruction of the conduct deluding karma. The aspirant concentrates upon the various aspects of reality. This type of meditation involves shifting of attention between the meaning, word and activity of the aspects of reality. Hence, it is called multi aspect meditation with shifting. This meditation suppresses or eliminates conduct deluding karma.

Single aspect spiritual meditation is contemplation on a single aspect of reality on the basis of scriptural knowledge by an aspirant who is in the delusion free (kshina moha) spiritual stage. The aspirant concentrates on one particular form or word or activity of the aspect of reality without shifting. Such meditation is the single aspect stage of spiritual meditation. This meditation eliminates the four destructive (ghatiya) karmas, namely, perception obscuring karma, knowledge obscuring karma, deluding karma and obstructing karma. Thus, it leads to omniscience.

Subtle activity spiritual meditation is performed by an omniscient who eliminates the gross activities of body, speech and mind, and possess only subtle activities. In such as case the association of soul with body causes only subtle movements of the space-points of the soul. Hence it is called the subtle activity stage of spiritual meditation.

Absorption in self-spiritual meditation is performed by an omniscient who eliminates even the slight activity of the soul in spite of its association with body. All activities (of the space-points of the soul) cease in this meditation. Thus the influx of even the pleasant feeling producing (sata vedaniya) karma is stopped. Finally all karmas are shed and the soul attains salvation. This is meditation according to Jain scriptures.

Yoga and Buddhism

Buddhist Philospohy

The Buddhist schools, of which there are four in classical Indian philosophy, though they share many ideas and with Vedic spirituality, like karma and rebirth, do not accept the authority of the Vedas and rejected certain key Vedic principles.

Buddhism has basically two varieties. The northern, Mahayana or "great vehicle" tradition, which prevails in Tibet, China and Japan and adjacent countries. This is the type of Buddhism that is most known and followed by the largest number of people. It includes Chan, Zen, Buddhist Tantra, Vajrayana, and Dzog Chen. The southern, Theravadin, prevails in the south of Asia, Sri Lanka, Burma and Thailand. Vipassana is the most commonly known practice of Theravada Buddhism. Generally the Theravadin form is considered to be the older of the two forms of Buddhism. However, most Indian Buddhism, including the Sanskrit Buddhist Sutras, is of the Mahayana branch and has been best preserved in Tibet, where it has undergone a further development into Vajrayana. There are some disagreements between these two main Buddhist lines philosophically.

The Mahayana tradition, particularly in its Tantric forms, uses breathing exercises, mantras, visualizations and deities much like the Yoga tradition. The Theravadin tradition has less in common with Yoga, though does use similar meditation and concentration methods. For example, some Vipassana teachers have often criticized the use of mantra, which is common not only in Hindu Yogic traditions but in the Mahayana Buddhist teachings.

Buddhism grew up in a cultural base of Hinduism. For this reason Indian and Tibetan Buddhism include Ayurvedic medicine, Hindu astrology, Sanskrit, the same rules of iconography and forms of temple worship, and other common factors as the Hindu tradition. A number of Hindu Gods and Goddesses, like Ganesha and Sarasvati, appear in the Buddhist tradition. Some figures like the Goddess Tara appear in both. Yet as Buddhism moved to other countries outside of India many of these connections were forgotten.

Nepal has remained as one country in which both these religions have continued, though Nepal has a Hindu majority, a Hindu king and has been officially a Hindu state. Yet in Nepal Hindu Yoga and Buddhists traditions are rarely simply equated. Nepalese Hindus and Buddhists respect one another but tend to follow one tradition but seldom both.

Similarities between Buddhist and Vedic Yoga

Yoga and Buddhism are both meditation traditions devised to help us transcend karma and rebirth and realize the truth of consciousness. They see the suffering and impermanence inherent in all birth and seek to alleviate it through developing a higher awareness. Both emphasize the need to dissolve the ego, the sense of the me and the mine, and return to the original reality that is not limited by the separate self. Both traditions emphasize enlightenment or inner illumination to be realized through meditation.

Both systems recognize dharma, the principle of truth or natural law, as the basic law of the universe we must come to understand. Such dharmas are the law of karma and the unity of all sentient beings. Buddhism defines itself as Buddha Dharma or the dharma of the enlightened ones, which is seen as a tradition transcending time or place. Yoga defines itself as part of the Hindu tradition called Sanatana Dharma, the universal or eternal dharma, which is not defined according to any particular teacher or tradition. Both traditions have called themselves Arya Dharma or the Dharma of the noble truth.

The main differences between the two systems are at a philosophical level, though both can be very diverse in this regard. Vedic systems are built upon fundamental principles like the Self (Atman), the Cosmic Lord (Ishvara), and Godhead or Absolute (Brahman). Buddhism tends to reject such ontological principles as creations of the mind itself. In this regard Vedic systems are more idealistic and Buddhism systems more phenomenological. Apart from such philosophical differences both systems share the same basic ethical values like non-violence, truthfulness, non-attachment and non-stealing. The vows that Buddhist monks take and those that monks and sadhus take in the Yoga tradition are the same, so are those of Jain monks.

The Absolute

Vedanta defines the absolute as a metaphysical principle Being-Consciousness-Bliss, or Brahman in which there is perfect peace and liberation. Buddhism does recognize an Absolute, which is non-dual and beyond all birth and death. However, Buddhism generally does not allow it any definition and regards it as Void or Shunyata. It is sometimes called the Dharmakaya or body of dharma.

Self and Not-Self

Buddhism generally rejects the Self (Atman or Purusha) of Yoga-Vedanta and emphasizes the non-Self (anatman). It says that there is no Self in anything and therefore that the Self is merely a fiction of the mind. Whatever we point out as the Self, the Buddhists state, is merely some impression, thought or feeling, but no such homogenous entity like a Self can be found anywhere.

The Yoga-Vedanta tradition emphasizes Self-realization or the realization of our true nature. It states that the Self does not exist in anything external. If we cannot find a self in anything it is no wonder, because if we did find a self in something it would not be the self but that particular thing. We cannot point out anything as the Self because the Self is the one who points all things out. The Self transcends the mind-body complex, but this is not to say that it does not exist. Without the Self we would not exist. We would not even be able to ask questions.

Yoga-Vedanta discriminates between the Self (Atman), which is our true nature as consciousness, and the ego (generally called ahamkara), which is the false identification of our true nature with the mind-body complex. The Atman of Vedanta is not the ego but is the enlightened awareness which transcends time and space. However a number of Buddhist traditions, particularly traditions outside of India, like the Chan and Zen traditions of China, have used terms like Self-mind, one's original nature, the original nature of consciousness or one's original face, which are similar to the Self of Vedanta.

Mind and Self

Buddhism defines reality in terms of mind and often refers to ultimate truth as the One Mind or original nature of the mind. In Yoga, mind (manas) is regarded as an instrument of consciousness that is the Self. It speaks of the One Self and the many minds which are its vehicles. For it mind is not an ultimate principle but something created.

If we examine the terms mind and Self in the two traditions it appears that what Yoga criticizes as attachment to the mind and ego is much like the Buddhist criticism of the attachment to the self, while what Yoga calls the Supreme Self or Purusha is similar to the Buddhist idea of the original nature of the Mind or One Mind. The Buddhist enlightened mind which dwells within the heart (Bodhicitta) resembles the Supreme

Self (Paramatman) which also dwells within the heart. Yet these similarities aside, the formulations and methodologies of the two systems can be quite different.

Ishvara or the Creator

The Yoga tradition is based upon a recognition of, respect for and devotion to God or the creator, preserver and dissolver of the universe. One of its main principles is surrender to God or the Divine within (Ishvara-Pranidhana), which is said to be the most direct method to Self-realization. Theism occurs in the various Yoga-Vedanta teachings, though often subordinated to the Self-Absolute, which transcends even the Creator. This is perhaps the main point of difference between Yoga and Buddhism. Buddhism rejects God (Ishvara) or a cosmic lord and creator. It sees no need for any creator and considers that living beings arise through karma alone. The Dalai Lama recently noted that Buddha is similar to God in omniscience but is not a creator of the universe.

Yet some modern Buddhist teachers use the term God and make it equivalent to the Buddha-nature. There is also the figure of the Adi-Buddha or primordial Buddha in some Buddhist traditions who resembles Ishvara. Lord Buddha appears as God not in the sense of a theological entity but as the Divine potential inherent in living being and is similarly is prayed to for forgiveness of misdeeds.

Karma and Rebirth

Both systems see karma as the main causative factor behind rebirth in the world. However, in Buddhism karma is said to be a self-existent principle. Buddhism states that the world exists owing to the beginningless karma of living beings. In Yoga and Vedanta, however, karma is not a self-existent principle. The world is created by God (Ishvara), the creative aspect of consciousness. Karma as a mere force of inertia and attachment cannot explain the creation of the world but only our attachment to it. Karma is a force dispensed by God, which cannot exist by itself, just as a lawcode cannot exist without a judge. However some other Vedic systems, also, like Purva Mimamsa put more emphasis upon karma than upon God or Ishvara.

Yoga recognizes the existence of a Jiva or individual soul who is reborn in various bodies. Buddhism denies the existence of such a soul and says that rebirth is just the continuance of a stream of karma, not any real entity.

Buddhist traditions go back to Lord Buddha and most emphasize studying the life of the historical Buddha, Shakyamuni. The Vedic tradition, on the other hand, recognizes many great teachers and avatars and there is no single teacher that everyone must follow or look back to. Hinduism has accepted Buddha as a great teacher but it has included him among its stream of many other teachers, gurus and avatars.

The term Buddha is common in Vedic teachings, as it is a common Sanskrit term meaning wise, awake, aware or enlightened. When Buddhism is referred to in Hindu literature it is usually called Bauddha Dharma or Saugata Dharma, as there is nothing in the term Buddha in Sanskrit that refers to a particular person or religion. While Hindus make Buddha into an avatar, in Buddhism Buddha cannot be an avatar because Buddhism has no God that Buddha could manifest.

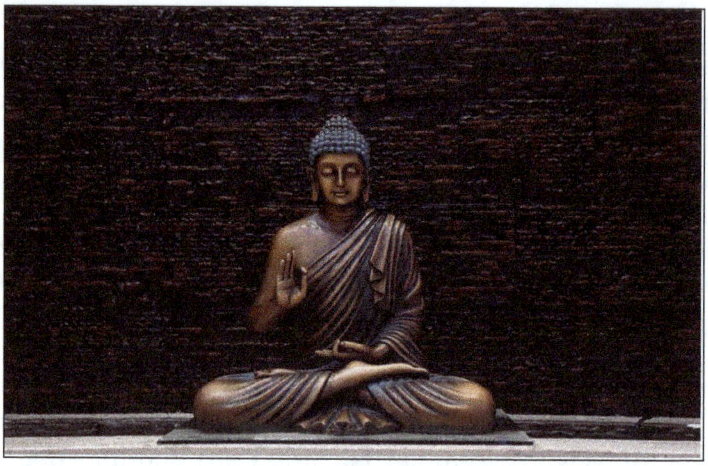

The Figure of the Buddha.

Nirvana

Both systems regard Nirvana or mergence in the Absolute as a primary goal of practice. However in the Buddhist tradition, Nirvana is generally described only negatively as cessation. It is given no positive appellations. In the Vedic tradition Nirvana is described in a positive way as mergence into Brahman or Sacchidananda, Being-Consciousness-Bliss, the realization of the infinite and eternal Self, called Brahma Nirvana. Yet both systems agree that this truth transcends all concepts. Vedanta describes Nirvana as freedom or liberation (Moksha). This term does not occur in Buddhism which does not accept the existence of any soul that can be liberated.

Devotion and Compassion

Yoga with its recognition of God emphasizes devotion and surrender to God (Ishvara-pranidhana) as one of the main spiritual paths. It contains an entire Yogic approach based on devotion, Bhakti Yoga, through which we open our hearts to God and surrender to the Divine Will. As Buddhism does not recognize God, devotion to God does not appear so clearly as a Buddhist path. Yet Buddhists do emphasize devotion to the Buddha and great Bodhisattvas and so does have a devotional component. Tibetan Buddhists have deity Yoga.

Buddhism emphasizes the role of the Bodhisattva, the enlightened one who stays on after enlightenment to teach and guide living beings. As according to Yoga the Divine and all the sages merged in it are ever present to help all beings, so there is no need for such a special Bodhisattva vow. Yoga values compassion as an ethical principle, however, and says that we cannot realize our true Self as long as we think that we are separate from other creatures.

Gods and Goddesses/Buddhas and Bodhisattvas

Buddhas and Bodhisattvas, therefore, are not deities or Gods and Goddesses. They are not forms of the Divine Father and Mother and have no role in creating, preserving and dissolving the universe. They are not the parents of all creatures but wise guides and teachers. They are described as great beings who once lived and attained enlightenment and took various vows to stay in the world to save living beings.

For example perhaps the greatest Buddhist Goddess, Tara is such a Bodhisattva, an enlightened person – not the Divine Mother like Durga or Kali of Hinduism – but a great enlightened sage who has continued to exist in the world. She is not the Goddess as the universal creator but an expression of the enlightened mind and its power of compassion. There are also meditation Buddhas (Dhyani Buddhas), who represent archetypes of enlightenment.

Yet though the Buddhas and Bodhisattvas are not forms of any Cosmic Creator, they can be prayed to for grace and protection. For example, the Bodhisattva Tara was thought to save those in calamities. Worship of various Bodhisattvas is called Deity Yoga in the Tibetan tradition.

Differences between Buddhist and Vedic Yoga

Buddhist texts, both Mahayana and Theravadin, contain refutations of the Atman, Brahman, Ishvara, and other key tenets of Hindu Yoga and Vedanta. Note the Lankavatara Sutra, which is typical in this regard. Refutation of Buddhist teachings does not occur in the Vedas, which are pre-Buddhist but do occur in later Hindu literature. Vedantic, Samkhya and Yoga texts contain refutations of several Buddhist doctrines. Criticisms of Buddhist teachings occur in the main commentaries on the Yoga Sutras, starting from that of Vyasa, and are common in Vedanta.

Such critiques can be found among the works of the greatest Hindu and Buddhist sages like Shankara of the Hindus, Nagarjuna and Aryadeva of the Buddhists. Relative to Yoga and Buddhism one of the most interesting interactions was between Ishvara Krishna (not Krishna of the Bhagavad Gita) and the Buddhist guru of Vasubandhu, the founder of the Vijnanavada school. The debate was said to be won by Ishvara Krishna and the record of his arguments, the Samkhya Karika was produced, which has become the main text on Samkhya. Vijnanavada, also called Yogachara, is perhaps the closest Buddhist school to classical Yoga, but curiously was the Buddhist system most in conflict with it in philosophical debates.

Yet we must note there have been similar debates within each tradition, with Advaita Vedanta critiques of other Hindu traditions like Samkhya-Yoga, or Buddhist Madhyamika critiques of Buddhist Vijnanavada and other Buddhist traditions. The Indian tradition cherished debate as a means of finding truth and did not simply aim at superficial intellectual agreements. This tradition of free and open debate is alive not only in India but in Tibet.

Buddhist Meditation

1. Samatha Meditation or Calm Abiding Meditation: This practice usually involves watching our breath as our object of meditation. This meditation is specifically designed to calm and focus our mind so we can develop our powers of concentration. We can also add a technique of counting our breaths to help increase our concentration and reduce the general distractibility of our mind. It is also possible to use an external object for this type of meditation. You might choose to meditate on a Buddha statue and place all your visual and mental attention on one aspect of it. Usually it's best to select a specific part of the statue to meditate on, rather than trying to focus on the whole thing. You could alternatively use a photo of the Buddha or your teacher to also inspire faith and devotion. Or you can just meditate on a small part of any object in front of you. I often focus on a small plastic blue flower, placing all my concentration on the center of it.

In the short term, this meditation will bring greater peace, happiness and clarity to your life if you practice it on a weekly or (better yet!) daily basis. But its main objective is to help establish a concentrated and stable mind so you can move onto the final goal of developing insight. When we can access deeper states of awareness, it will reveal the true nature of ourselves and our reality which leads to ultimate peace and happiness (Awakening/Enlightenment).

Variations: There are a number of variations we can make to the common practice of watching our breath, especially if our mind is particularly distracted or distressed by negative emotions.

- Adding colors to your breath if you're a visual person.
- Adding qualities to the breath to help remove negative emotions, for instance, visualizing you're breathing in a positive quality and breathing out something negative that you need to let go of.

2. Walking Meditation: Not all of us are great at sitting for long periods of time. Fortunately, we can break up our sessions with walking meditation. At full day retreats, it is common to interchange sitting and walking meditations so that one hour of sitting meditation is followed by 30 minutes of walking meditation. Generally, walking meditation is designed to complement our sitting meditations so that we maintain our concentration between our seated sessions. This meditation pays close attention to the movement of our feet as we walk slowly, back and forth, in a small, defined area.

Developing Wisdom and Insight (Enlightenment)

- Vipassana Meditation: This meditation involves paying attention to the arising and passing away of sensations in each of your different parts of your body. In Theravada Buddhist schools, this is the pinnacle of meditation practices, being the main method for developing insight into our true nature. Notably, most Theravada schools will always incorporate some sort of samatha practice before moving onto Vipassana meditation. Other Buddhist schools similarly practice Vipassana, although it can sometimes take a more analytical approach of questioning, such as 'where is the Self?', and through examination one becomes free from self-grasping.

- Koans: These are usually a phrase or question that a meditator repeatedly brings to mind. It is not solvable through conceptual thinking and it attempts to push the meditator's mind into an experience beyond thought. It is believed that shortcutting the intellectual process can lead to direct realisation. A well-known koan is 'what is your original face before you were born?'

- Shikantaza ("just sitting"): This is an objectless meditation where the aim is to simply remain in a state of concentration of the act of sitting while simultaneously being aware of what arises in your mind. Different schools might have different approaches, but if insight isn't gained from koan practice, then generally the powerful concentration developed first from breathing meditation or koans can allow insight to arise in Shikantaza where one can see the arising and passing away of all phenomena in every moment.

Developing Loving-Kindness and Compassion

- Metta (Loving-Kindness) Meditation: This meditation aims at increasing our feeling of loving-kindness to everyone. We first practice generating metta (wishing others happiness) by meditating on objects that are easiest to arouse loving-kindness for. Then we progressively move to more difficult objects of metta, like our enemies. This practice is an effective technique for eliminating our hatred and anger towards others.

- Meditation on the Sameness of Self and Others: This meditation aims at highlighting our shared humanity and that no one wants to experience suffering. By putting ourselves in others' shoes, it can increase our compassion for everyone regardless of who they are.

- Tonglen Meditation: Tonglen means 'giving and receiving'. Here we imagine that we're taking on the suffering of others and giving them all the things they need to alleviate their suffering. This practice is sometimes known as 'the secret' and is powerful in increasing our compassion and reducing our selfishness and self-grasping.

Analytical Meditations to Enhance the Buddha's Teachings

- Meditation on the Faults of Samsara: This meditation looks at the multitude of sufferings that sentient beings can experience in the world. Most importantly, it focuses the various sufferings that human beings can experience. Although this meditation helps to develop compassion for others, its primarily aim is to highlight that external worldly aims (like having money, fame and nice possessions) do not bring ever-lasting happiness. It reminds us that happiness is to be found within, not from external phenomena. This meditation is particularly helpful to strengthen our renunciation and to help us stay committed to our meditation practice, lest we get lost in pursing the ephemeral, unsatisfactory pleasures of the world.

- Meditation on our Precious Human Life: According to the Buddha, gaining a human rebirth is extremely rare. Moreover, gaining a human life that has the necessary conditions for being able to practice his teachings is rarer still! This meditation focuses on how difficult it is to obtain this human life so we can appreciate the opportunity we have now to practice.

- Meditation on Impermanence: This meditation closely ties in with the previous one. When we truly realize how short our time on Earth is, it will inspire us to practice NOW and not procrastinate. Also, when we really feel this law of impermanence in our bones, we will accept the changing aspects of our life more readily so we can let go of things (and people) more easily, as everything is destined to change.

- Meditation on Equanimity: Often we easily define people in our life into categories: those we love, hate or feel indifferent towards. According to the Buddha, these are all delusions; we shouldn't fix permanent labels to ever-changing phenomena. This meditation helps us to break down the labels we've given people in our lives, so we can develop loving-kindness and compassion equally to all.

- Meditation on Remembering the Kindness of Mother Sentient Beings: The aim of this meditation is to remind us of the kindness of our mothers so we can develop a heart of gratitude. It also helps us develop a sense of responsibility to repay their kindness, not just to them but to all sentient beings that have presumably been our mothers in a past life. This practice is extremely powerful in combating any aversion we might have to our present-life mother.

- Meditation on the Impurities of our Bodies: This meditation is specifically designed to combat our lust and craving for sexual encounters. Traditionally, the Buddha taught this technique to celibate monks to try and help curb their sexual impulses and keep their mind on the task of one-pointed meditation and reaching nirvana. This meditation goes through all the parts of the body in all its wonderful gross detail, so we can really acknowledge what the human body is made up of (e.g. blood, skin, pus and hair). By doing this we won't be so quick to exaggerate physical beauty and can see the human form in a more balanced way.

Meditations to Allay Meditative Obstacles and Quicken One's Realization of Emptiness

Deity Meditations

Vajrayana Buddhism (also known as Tibetan Buddhism) and many Mahayana Buddhist schools are filled with a multitude of deity meditation practices. These sometimes involve visualizing the deity as an external being that we can request blessings from. But the real transformative meditations are the ones where you visualize yourself as the deity, in their form, reciting their mantras, and meditating on the spiritual qualities they possess (immeasurable compassion and wisdom). Through the power of imagining yourself as the 'end result' – as a being that's already enlightened – we can help those qualities to germinate and come to fruition faster. These meditations also help break us free of clinging to self, as we're no longer identifying with our ordinary, egoistic self, but rather one who is endowed with enlightened qualities.

There are literally hundreds of different deity meditation practices and each school has practices which they favor most, so it's impossible to list them all. But below we have listed some of the more common deity practices found in most of the Vajrayana Buddhist schools and some of their specific purposes.

- Green Tara: Seen as the female embodiment of all the Buddha's wisdom, she is considered the mother who dispels all fears.
- Chenrezig (4 or 1000 armed): The Buddha of compassion. Meditating on him increases our compassion for all sentient beings without discrimination. In the female form, he appears as Quan Yin, especially in Chinese Buddhist schools.
- Medicine Buddha: Meditating on his form and mantra increases our compassion and can bring healing to ourselves and others.
- Vajrasattva: Recognized to be the superior of all the practices to help purify our negative karma.
- White Tara: She is another form of Tara, but her meditation is designed specifically to increase our lifespan so we can continue to practice Dharma and help others.

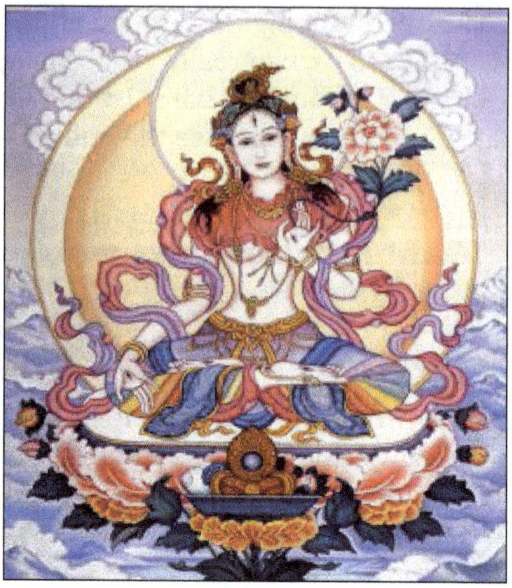

White Tara.

References

- What-you-may-not-realize-about-yoga: yogainternational.com, Retrieved 10, May 2020
- Transcendental-Meditation: lakshminarayanlenasia.com, Retrieved 25, July 2020
- How-do-I-perform-Transcendental-Meditation: quora.com, Retrieved 18, February 2020
- Yoga-and-meditation-in-jainism: blogspot.com, Retrieved 09, June 2020
- The-meaning-of-yoga-according-to-jain-philosophy: veerayatan.org, Retrieved 14, April 2020
- Yoga-and-buddhism-similarities-and-differences: vedanet.com, Retrieved 26, January 2020
- 15-best-meditation-techniques-buddhism-beginners-advanced: enthusiasticbuddhist.com, Retrieved 17, March 2020
- Mahasi-sayadaw-1951-practical-vipassana-meditation-exercises: saraniya.com, Retrieved 21, August 2020

Permissions

All chapters in this book are published with permission under the Creative Commons Attribution Share Alike License or equivalent. Every chapter published in this book has been scrutinized by our experts. Their significance has been extensively debated. The topics covered herein carry significant information for a comprehensive understanding. They may even be implemented as practical applications or may be referred to as a beginning point for further studies.

We would like to thank the editorial team for lending their expertise to make the book truly unique. They have played a crucial role in the development of this book. Without their invaluable contributions this book wouldn't have been possible. They have made vital efforts to compile up to date information on the varied aspects of this subject to make this book a valuable addition to the collection of many professionals and students.

This book was conceptualized with the vision of imparting up-to-date and integrated information in this field. To ensure the same, a matchless editorial board was set up. Every individual on the board went through rigorous rounds of assessment to prove their worth. After which they invested a large part of their time researching and compiling the most relevant data for our readers.

The editorial board has been involved in producing this book since its inception. They have spent rigorous hours researching and exploring the diverse topics which have resulted in the successful publishing of this book. They have passed on their knowledge of decades through this book. To expedite this challenging task, the publisher supported the team at every step. A small team of assistant editors was also appointed to further simplify the editing procedure and attain best results for the readers.

Apart from the editorial board, the designing team has also invested a significant amount of their time in understanding the subject and creating the most relevant covers. They scrutinized every image to scout for the most suitable representation of the subject and create an appropriate cover for the book.

The publishing team has been an ardent support to the editorial, designing and production team. Their endless efforts to recruit the best for this project, has resulted in the accomplishment of this book. They are a veteran in the field of academics and their pool of knowledge is as vast as their experience in printing. Their expertise and guidance has proved useful at every step. Their uncompromising quality standards have made this book an exceptional effort. Their encouragement from time to time has been an inspiration for everyone.

The publisher and the editorial board hope that this book will prove to be a valuable piece of knowledge for students, practitioners and scholars across the globe.

Index

A

Anulom Vilom, 143-149, 180-181, 183

Ashtanga Yoga, 36, 115, 125, 196

Assimilation, 165

B

Baddha Konasana, 13, 30

Balasana, 11, 18, 60

Base Chakra, 144

Bhakti Yoga, 2-3, 44, 52-54, 58, 120, 228

Bhramari, 149-151, 154, 190

Bhujangasana, 33, 105, 164, 172

Blood Pressure, 137, 139, 142, 145, 147, 153, 166, 173, 185, 204-205, 207

Brahmacharya, 37, 118

C

Capillary Action, 159

Cardiovascular Endurance, 6

Chakras, 4, 67-68, 74-81, 84-85, 88, 97-98, 108, 114, 186

Chakrasana, 164

Composition, 134, 166

Computer Programmers, 195

Conceptualization, 63

Confucianism, 113

Conjunction, 105, 194

Consciousness, 1, 4, 37, 39, 42, 45, 58, 61, 63, 71, 77, 79-82, 114, 120, 125-126, 192, 195, 198, 203, 207, 212, 218, 220, 225-228

Cookies, 50

Corpse Pose, 32, 102

Crown Chakra, 77, 80-81, 144

D

Dakshina Nauli, 167, 170, 172

Dhanurasana, 35, 105

Dharana, 36, 39, 126, 131, 192

Dhauti, 156, 163-166

Dhyana Mudra, 109

Digital Library, 105

E

Endocrine System, 80-81, 83

Etymology, 74, 114, 118, 123, 126

F

Facial Expressions, 106

Fatigue, 103, 138, 146, 149, 157, 180, 204, 209

G

Gene Expression, 117

Gestures, 108, 112

H

Hatha Yoga, 3-4, 40-41, 44, 52, 67, 102, 104-106, 114, 117, 119-121, 132, 140-141, 156-158, 166-167, 171, 173, 176, 185

Hatha Yoga Pradipika, 105-106, 114, 117, 119-121, 132, 156-157, 166, 171, 173

Hrid Dhauti, 166

Hyperactivity, 7

I

Ida, 68, 82, 97

Interpolation, 115

Introspection, 45, 120, 209, 215

Iyengar Yoga, 104

J

Jala Basti, 171-173

P

Physical Activities, 221

Pingala Nadi, 97

Plethora, 93

Potential Energy, 64

Power Yoga, 41, 148

Pranayama, 2, 18, 36, 38, 41, 51, 58, 64, 101, 105, 126, 129, 148, 153, 157, 164, 172, 176, 191, 193, 208, 210

Pratyahara, 36, 38-39, 61, 125-127, 131, 208

Q

Qigong, 77

R
Raja Yoga, 3, 36, 52, 67, 120, 196
Ripple Effect, 107
Root Chakra, 5, 84

S
Sahasrara, 4, 81, 98, 184
Samadhi, 36, 39, 61, 81, 98, 126, 131, 184, 192, 196, 199, 218
Samkhya, 67, 70, 125, 229
Self-discipline, 36, 38, 40, 120, 216, 221
Shankhaprakshalana, 164
Soft Palate, 113
Spiritual Development, 38, 217, 221
Spiritual Energy, 217
Squatting, 163
Sthula Sarira, 67, 70, 72
String, 30, 130, 161
Surya Namaskar, 59
Sushumna, 68, 75, 81-82, 97, 131, 141, 144
Svadhishthana, 5, 84
Svadhyaya, 38, 42, 44, 120, 123
Syllables, 79, 116
Sympathetic Nervous System, 62, 97

T
Tadasana, 59, 164
Tantra Yoga, 2, 58, 60
Tapas, 117, 119-120, 123, 194-195
Transcendental Meditation, 195-199, 203, 206-208
Trataka, 39, 156, 185-186, 189, 191-193
Turiya, 46, 71

U
Uddiyana Bandha, 167-168, 172
Ujjayi, 140, 150, 185
Ujjayi Pranayama, 140, 150, 185
Uttanasana, 9, 59

V
Vajrasana, 17-18, 105-107, 140, 164, 179-180
Vatsara Dhauti, 163
Vedanta, 3, 67, 69, 71-72, 124-125, 226-229
Viniyoga, 41
Vinyasa Yoga, 102, 104
Vipassana Meditation, 231
Visuddha, 82

W
Walking Meditation, 230

Y
Yoga Physiology, 71
Yoga Sutra, 2, 102, 104
Yogic Breathing, 105

www.ingramcontent.com/pod-product-compliance
Lightning Source LLC
LaVergne TN
LVHW080625210926
848485LV00003B/211